Professional Practice in Paramedic, Emergency and Urgent Care

Professional Practice in Paramedic, Emergency and Urgent Care

Edited by

Val Nixon
MSc, BSc (Hons), RN (DipN) London

Academic Group Lead for Adult Nursing
Faculty of Health Sciences
Staffordshire University
UK

⟨W⟩WILEY-BLACKWELL

A John Wiley & Sons, Ltd., Publication

This edition first published 2013
© 2013 by John Wiley & Sons, Ltd

Registered office: John Wiley & Sons, Ltd, The Atrium, Southern Gate, Chichester,
West Sussex, PO19 8SQ, UK

Editorial offices: 9600 Garsington Road, Oxford, OX4 2DQ, UK
The Atrium, Southern Gate, Chichester, West Sussex, PO19 8SQ, UK
111 River Street, Hoboken, NJ 07030-5774, USA

For details of our global editorial offices, for customer services and for information about how to apply
for permission to reuse the copyright material in this book please see our website at
www.wiley.com/wiley-blackwell.

Library of Congress Cataloging-in-Publication Data

Professional practice in paramedic, emergency, and urgent care / edited by Val Nixon.
    p. ; cm.
  Includes bibliographical references and index.
  ISBN 978-0-470-65615-0 (pbk. : alk. paper) – ISBN 978-1-118-48818-8 (emobi) –
  ISBN 978-1-118-48822-5 (epub) – ISBN 978-1-118-48823-2 (epdf)
  I. Nixon, Val.
  [DNLM: 1. Emergency Medical Services–Great Britain.   2. Allied Health Personnel–Great Britain.
3. Ambulatory Care–Great Britain.   4. Clinical Competence–Great Britain.   5. Nurses–Great
Britain.   WX 215]
  362.18–dc23
                                                                                    2012047810

A catalogue record for this book is available from the British Library.

Wiley also publishes its books in a variety of electronic formats. Some content that appears in print may
not be available in electronic books.

Cover image: © iStockphoto.com/PeskyMonkey
Cover design by Sarah Dickinson

Set in 9.5/12.5pt Palatino by Aptara® Inc., New Delhi, India
Printed and bound in Malaysia by Vivar Printing Sdn Bhd

1   2013

Contents

List of Contributors

Editor

Val Nixon, MSc, BSc (Hons), RN (DipN) London, Registered Nurse Teaching (RNT)

Val is a registered nurse and an Academic Group Leader for Adult Nursing in the Faculty of Health Sciences at Staffordshire University. Her previous role at Staffordshire University was a Principal Lecturer for Acute and Emergency Care which included paramedic education. Val started her career in Emergency Nursing and took up a variety of roles including Emergency Nurse Practitioner and Clinical Educator and in 2004 she moved into Higher Education to begin her teaching career at Staffordshire University. Val has an MSc in Professional Education, a BSc (Hons) in Nursing Studies and has recently commenced a PhD at Staffordshire University. Val has also worked for the West Midlands NHS Strategic Health Authority and Skills for Health to undertake several projects for the non-medical staff working in emergency and urgent care. This included roles, skills and competences against the national career framework and educational development needs. She is currently leading on a project to work towards developing a regional mentor framework for the West Midlands region in collaboration with the regional ambulance service and other universities who provide paramedic education in the West Midlands.

Contributors

Matt Capsey, BSc (Hons), PgC, MCPara

Matt is a paramedic and Senior Lecturer in Paramedic Science at Teesside University having previously worked in practice in North Yorkshire. He holds a Bachelor's Degree in Sociology and Social Psychology, Postgraduate Certificate in Learning and Teaching in Higher Education and is completing a Master's Degree in Paramedic Science at the University of Hertfordshire. He has previously represented the Northeast region on the national governing council of the College of Paramedics and chaired the regional group.

Karen Gubbins, MSc, BSC, PgC, BSc (Hons), MCPara, FHEA

Karen is a paramedic and a Senior Lecturer for paramedic programmes at Worcester University. Karen joined the ambulance service in 1996, and registered as a paramedic in 1998. She began her career in education within the ambulance service in 2002, and joined the University in 2007. She has a BSc in Applied Professional Studies, Postgraduate Certificate in Teaching and Learning and an MSc in Advanced Practice. Karen is currently a fellow member of the Higher Education Academy and has co-authored books on reflection.

Karen Latcham, MA (Keele) Medical Ethics and Law, Cert Ed (FAHE), RODP

Karen is a Senior Lecturer at Staffordshire University within Operating Department Practice education. Karen has worked within the perioperative environment in both NHS and independent sector since qualifying in 1991. She gained experience within the three areas of perioperative care, mentoring, assessment, clinical management and clinical effectiveness facilitation. She moved into full-time education in 2004 where she currently works as the Award Leader for the Operating Department Practice programme and manages and teaches several modules within the award. Karen has a Masters in Medical Ethics and Law and her teaching interests are anaesthetics, recovery, medical law and ethics. She links closely with clinical placement areas and supports student operating department practitioners whilst in clinical placement. Karen is an active member of the Interprofessional Working Group and works with colleagues across the faculty of health that facilitates a programme of interprofessional education for students of all disciplines.

Jacqui Mason, PGCIIPE, MSc, Dip NLP, PRINCE II, BSc (Hons), Higher Award A&E, RGN, RMN

Jacqui is a Senior Lecturer in Emergency Care at the Faculty of Health Sciences at Staffordshire University. Prior to joining the University, she has held a wide variety of clinical, managerial and teaching roles and is experienced in teaching different disciplines including postgraduate and undergraduate nurses, doctors and paramedics. In her current role, she works mainly with aspiring paramedics as the Award Leader for the Foundation Degree in Paramedic Science. Jacqui also leads on an Assessment and Management of Minor Injuries Module and a Risk, Decision Making and Uncertainty Module; as well as teaching on a wide variety of undergraduate and postgraduate awards. She continues to work in clinical practice within the Emergency Department and has commenced working towards her Professional Doctorate.

Lorna McInulty, MN (Master of Nursing), PGCHeRP, ONC (Orthopaedic Nursing Certificate), A/E Cert, FHEA, RGN

Lorna has many years of experience as an emergency nurse and was appointed one of the UK's first consultant nurses in 2001. Prior to this, she held a number of clinical teaching roles and is very experienced in teaching different disciplines including postgraduate and undergraduate nurses, doctors and paramedics. She has also been an active researcher. In her present role of Senior Lecturer in Emergency and Urgent Care at the University of Central Lancashire, she works mainly with aspiring paramedics but also contributes to a number of post-registration specialist courses for nurses working in emergency care. She holds a Master of Nursing degree from the University of Glasgow (1996) and was awarded a Postgraduate Certificate in Higher Education Research and Practice from the University of Salford (2007), with distinction. She is a registered nurse teacher with the Nursing and Midwifery Council and also a Fellow of the Higher Education Academy.

Kay Norman, MSc, PgD, BSc (Hons), PGDPHE, RGN

Kay is a Principal Lecturer in Community Based Care at the Faculty of Health Sciences at Staffordshire University. She is a registered nurse teacher with the Nursing and Midwifery Council and currently leads on a variety of community-based care educational programmes and has a particular interest in practice nursing, image of nursing, and leadership. Her current doctoral thesis concerns the exploration of young people's perceptions of nursing and the influences that have helped shape their views. Kay also works part time as a contraception and sexual health nurse within Royal Wolverhampton Hospitals Trust.

Louise Perkinton, MSc, BSc (Hons) Nursing Sciences, RN, DipAdEd, Registered Nurse Teacher, FHEA

Louise works as a Senior Lecturer at Derby University and is the programme leader on the pre-registration nursing degree and leads and teaches on evidence based practice module within this curriculum. She has been a nurse teacher for 20 years, working across a range of pre- and post-registration programmes in three Universities. Her teaching interests lie in research, critical care nursing and interprofessional education. Prior to moving into education, she was a ward sister in medical high dependency/coronary care. She holds a Master's degree in healthcare policy and organisation and she is a Fellow of the Higher Education Academy.

Introduction

Health policy changes from 1997 set out to modernise the NHS through the delivery and continuous improvements of high-quality healthcare services that was designed around the patients. As a result, demand-driven, high-profile services such as emergency and urgent care, saw the implementation of national standards to reduce waiting times and improve access to emergency and urgency care services. This led to dramatic changes in new ways of working, role redesign and changes in skill mix to redesign service delivery. Like the NHS, ambulance services in England are also playing an increasingly wide role in the NHS in response to national policy changes.

Traditionally, ambulance services have been designed around delivering resuscitation, trauma care and cardiac care to patients who are critically ill. Eighty percent of training to front-line ambulance clinicians has been focused on this. Today, 90% of patients do not fit into this category. Ambulance services have changed their traditional approach and are now more embedded in urgent care as a whole to provide a mobile healthcare service for the NHS. Added to this is an increase in public expectations, advanced medical and information technology, an ageing population and chronic conditions has put even greater pressure and demand on emergency and urgent care services. This has been a positive move towards roles of nurses and paramedics, perhaps politically driven but also out of the desire to enhance patient care, improve access, reduce unnecessary attendance to emergency departments, provide care closer to home and unlock and utilise nursing and paramedical potential.

The current provision of emergency and urgent care services, roles and responsibilities of nurses and paramedics are continuously evolving and increasing in the UK. Patients are now accessing and seeking care at the point of delivery. As a result, the front-line practitioners have to consider options for referral and the use of alternative care pathways. Paramedics and nurses working in this sector need to be educated and trained to deal with the mixed case they see both at the pre-registration education and continuing professional development. They must have the underpinning knowledge and skills which will enable the correct clinical decisions to be made, which are demonstrably in the patients' best interest. This can only be achieved in a clinically safe, professional and lawful manner (Nursing and Midwifery Council 2008; Health & Care Professions Council 2012).

This book is intended to provide the underpinning theoretical knowledge of the issues that you encounter on a daily basis when working in the pre-hospital, emergency and urgent care environment. This will hopefully enable you to develop a comprehensive theoretical understanding of the issues underpinning professional practice which is fundamental to everyday clinical practice. The chapters will provide clinical exemplars, discussion points and critical thinking points throughout. This is intended for you to reflect on your own experiences in order for you to link and apply the theory to your own area of practice. Illustrations given will also demonstrate how the theory is applied in practice to increase your understanding of the concepts explored in this book.

The first three chapters are focused on patient assessment which includes history taking, consultation and communication skills and clinical decision making. These three chapters are inextricably linked and cannot be viewed as separate subjects. Therefore, all three chapters should be read in conjunction with each other in order for you to gain a comprehensive theoretical understanding that will enable to justify your decision making when assessing and managing patient care.

For the remaining chapters, it is inevitable that the subject areas discussed and explored in this book are integrated with each other and therefore there will be some overlap in each individual chapter. Wherever possible, these have been cross-referenced to chapters where it is discussed more in detail.

As the book title suggests, it is intended for paramedics and nurses working in pre-hospital, emergency and urgent care. Chapters 3, 6 and 7 predominately focus on paramedic practice; however, the principles of professional practice are transferable and therefore can be applied to all areas of healthcare practice.

Paramedics and paramedic practice is an emerging profession and therefore the literature predominately relates to the clinical aspects of practice with very little relating to the professional aspect of practice. Therefore, the literature used throughout this book has been drawn from other disciplines, predominately nursing. It is important to understand that regardless of this, the theoretical knowledge and skills are transferable and will apply to all healthcare practitioners.

It is hoped that this book will enable you to develop a broader and deeper knowledge base of the theoretical issues that underpin professional practice and how this is applied to everyday clinical practice. I hope you enjoy reading this book as much as I have enjoyed writing and editing this book.

Val Nixon

References

Health & Care Professions Council (2012) *Code of Conduct, Performance and Ethics*. HCPC, London.

Nursing and Midwifery Council (2008) *The Code: Standards of Conduct, Performance and Ethics for Nurses and Midwives*. NMC, London.

Acknowledgements

I would like to say a huge thank you to all of the contributory authors for their valuable time and expertise in writing their chapters.

I also wish to say a big thank you to my colleagues, clinical mentors, nurses, paramedics and paramedic students who have taken the time to offer support, guidance and reviewing of chapters – your constructive comments and views have been extremely valuable.

A very huge thank you to my daughter, Natalie, who has been very patient and understanding over the many months I have spent writing this book. Thank you, my angel.

Val Nixon

1 History Taking

Val Nixon

Faculty of Health Sciences, Staffordshire University, Stafford, UK

Introduction

History taking is the critical first step in detecting the aetiology of a patient's problem using a systematic approach. Historically, history taking has been the domain of the medical practitioner whilst other professions focused on assessment skills related to particular body systems, or on assessing activities of daily living (ADL) such as communication, eating and drinking, washing and dressing. In recent years, professional boundaries between different healthcare professionals have begun to blur in response to healthcare reform. Subsequently, history taking skills are becoming increasingly important to non-medical healthcare professionals (Kaufman, 2008) and arguably the most important aspect of patient assessment (Crumbie, 2006). History taking should be clear and all elements should be conducted in the same way with the same purpose; to inform patient care, provide clear communication to other professions and prevent repetition and omission of relevant data. This chapter will therefore focus on the history, taking process using the medical model to structure this process. A brief introduction of why history taking is important will be offered followed by tools and mnemonics that you can use to support and guide your questioning techniques when obtaining information. There will be reference to the importance of communication skills needed when taking a patient's history; however, due to the complexity of this subject area, this has been explored fully in Chapter 2.

Obtaining the information

History taking is a process whereby the patient or others familiar with the patient report relevant complaints (subjective data) referred to as symptoms. Symptoms and clinical signs are ascertained by direct examination (objective data) by the healthcare professional. History taking is like

Professional Practice in Paramedic, Emergency and Urgent Care, First Edition. Edited by Val Nixon.
© 2013 John Wiley & Sons, Ltd. Published 2013 by John Wiley & Sons, Ltd.

playing detective; searching for clues, collecting information without bias, yet staying on track to solve the puzzle (Clarke, 1999). Essential and active listening skills are required and this is described by Duffy (1999) as the most fundamental communication skill and is central to obtaining a history. An accurate history can provide 80% or more of the information required for diagnosis (Epstein et al., 2008; Bickley and Szilagyi, 2009). The clinical examination and/or diagnostic testing should only confirm or disprove this diagnosis.

Medical histories vary in their depth and focus from case to case and according to their purpose. The medical history has a traditional format (see Box 1.1) which is considered the 'gold standard' (Bickley and Szilagyi, 2009). This provides a systematic approach, yet will generally require a flexible attitude and questioning techniques as opposed to a rigid interrogation or a checklist of questions.

Box 1.1   Traditional medical history

Date and time
Identifying data
Presenting complaint
History of presenting complaint
Past medical history
    Previous illness and surgery
    Drug history
    Allergies
Family history
Social history
Mental health history
Review of systems

There will be circumstances where a comprehensive history is required such as:

- Where reaching the diagnosis is difficult or complex
- Where the patient has a range of different health problems
- When the patient is a new patient in the hospital/GP setting
- Baseline for future assessments

Otherwise, there will be circumstances where the history should be more selective which is described as a focused history (Rushforth, 2009). Selected questions are directed towards the presenting problem or need may be more appropriate such as:

- Emergency situations where it is necessary to undertake a primary survey

- Minor illness or information where the information can focus directly to the patients' problem
- General mental health assessment

Irrespective of which approach is used, the history-taking process allows patients to present their account of the problem and provides essential information for the healthcare professional. It provides the opportunity for the patient to tell their story with an unfolding of symptoms, problems and feelings. It is important to recognise that patients tell their stories in different and usually unstructured ways which may lead to necessary information being omitted. It is, therefore, imperative for the practitioner to use effective communication skills within a systematic framework (see Chapter 2). This will prevent information being overlooked that is essential for diagnostic accuracy. There are several systematic frameworks to support the history-taking process. AMPLE (see Box 1.2) is advantageous for situations where depth and focus of the history are based on the case at hand. It is quick and easy to use especially in an emergency situation. A disadvantage of this framework is the lack of enough detail and structure to enable generation of a patient's condition, especially when asking events leading up to the emergency. Subsequently, the potential to miss out relevant questions is possible.

Box 1.2   AMPLE survey

Allergies
Medication/drug history
Past medical history
Last meal or oral intake
Events leading up to the emergency

Identifying the data

Start the history-taking process by identifying the age, sex, occupation and marital status of the patient. This will become important through other sections of this process. This source of information is generally obtained from the patient, but can also be obtained from a family member, friend or from a written source. Where appropriate, it is important to identify and record the source of information, as the accuracy of information obtained may be questionable. The patient's mood, memory, trust and clinical condition may affect the reliability of information given and these factors must also be identified and recorded.

The presenting complaint

Normally, the presenting complaint (PC) may only consist of two signs and symptoms; for example, 'chest pain', 'ankle injury' and 'feeling unwell' are initially reported and recorded. A range of differential diagnosis will be considered at this point of the history taking process. It is important to gather further information to eliminate some of the differential diagnosis and consider causes as to why the patient has sought medical assistance (Gregory and Murcell, 2010).

History of presenting complaint

This section of the process is the main component of history taking. A detailed and thorough investigation into the current illness is performed to provide a complete, clear and chronological account for the PC(s) prompting the patient to seek care. This usually comprises two sequential (but overlapping) stages:

- The patient's account of the symptoms
- Specific, detailed questions by the health professional undertaking the history

To obtain the patient's account of symptoms, the use of open-ended questions is required. This is to avoid a yes or no answer so that the patient can expand on their story. For example, 'tell me more about your chest pain' encourages the patient to tell the practitioner more. In contrast, closed questions such as 'is the chest pain severe?' can be answered in a 'yes' or 'no,' which is useful for seeking specific answers that are required to gain a deeper understanding of the patient's problem (Kaufman, 2008).

It is important to listen to patients as they tell you their story as generally they are telling you their diagnosis. Listening should be an active process and patients should be given every opportunity to talk freely at the start of the consultation with minimal interruption (Marsh, 1999). A common mistake is for the health professional to intervene too early, and research has shown the importance of listening to patients' opening statements without interruption (Gask and Usherwood, 2002). Once a patient has been interrupted, they rarely introduce new issues (Gask and Usherwood, 2002) and vital information may never come to light (Kaufman, 2008). If uninterrupted, most patients will tell you their problem in 1–2 minutes (Snadden et al., 2005). It is a matter of judgement when to start interrupting and asking open questions, but as a general rule, think twice before interrupting a patient in full flow as this may not be what is concerning the patient the most. A combination of art, experience and patience determines when and how to interrupt a patient in full flow and every attempt to use the patient's own words is essential. Remember the most important facts given by the patient as these may need further clarification.

Once the patient has given their account of the signs and symptoms of the presenting problem, closed questions may be used to focus on gathering information that is relevant to the history of the presenting complaint (HPC). A chronological account of the symptoms and associated symptoms should be explored in a systematic manner, and include onset of the problem, the setting in which it has developed, its manifestations and any therapeutic interventions used to relieve symptoms (Bickley and Szilagyi, 2009). The use of a mnemonic can provide a systematic approach so that a single event or system can be explored more fully and consequently encourage patients to expand and describe their symptoms. One mnemonic is the OPQRST (Morton, 1993). This mnemonic is mostly used in describing pain but can also be used as a symptom analysis (see Box 1.3). Other mnemonics which can be used are illustrated in Boxes 1.4 and 1.5.

Box 1.3   OPQRST mnemonic

O onset
P provocative/palliative
Q quality
R region/radiation
S severity
T temporal/timing

Box 1.4   TROCARSS mnemonic

T timing
R rapidity
O occurrence
C characteristics
A associations
R relief
S site
S spread
S severity

Box 1.5   SOCRATES mnemonic

S site
O onset
C character . . . sharp, dull
R radiation
A alleviating factors
T timing
E exacerbating factors
S severity 1–10

Onset

It is important to determine when the symptom/pain started as this is a key factor to determine whether it is acute, chronic, urgent or non-urgent. Establishing the speed of onset to determine the rate of development (seconds, minutes, hours etc.) is useful too. Start with open-ended questions such as 'what were you doing when this started?' or 'do you have a history of this problem?' or 'when did you last feel well?' It is important not to ask leading questions that may elicit the wrong response. For example, 'did it start yesterday?' or 'were you active at the time?'

Provocative/palliative

Questions relating to what provoked the symptom/pain; and any medication either prescribed over the counter or herbal/homeopathic or other alternatives that made the symptom/pain better or worse should be considered. Factors such as movement, lying down, sitting up, on rest, on exertion and breathing should also be considered as this is important towards confirming or disproving differential diagnosis. For example, a patient complaining of left-sided chest pain lasting for several minutes that developed following an exertion or emotional stress (provocative factors) and/or relieved by rest or Glyceryl Trinitrate (palliative) may be indicative of unstable angina, whereas persistent chest pain that may not have provocative factors and is unresponsive to palliative measures may be indicative of unstable angina or myocardial infarction.

Quality

Patients will use a variety of words to describe their symptoms; and prompting the patients to define this symptom is particularly useful in arriving at a diagnosis (Crumbie, 2006). For example, crushing chest pain is almost diagnostic of myocardial infarction. Throbbing, burning, hot, heavy, stabbing, sharp, shooting, tender are various other descriptions patients may use to describe their discomfort.

Region/radiation

Discovering where the symptom/pain is being experienced is fundamental as it often gives clues to the aetiology. This may be a vague description by the patient as the patient may describe the region more broadly, for example, 'pain in my stomach'. As there are several structures within the abdominal cavity, it would be difficult to identify the exact nature of the problem. It is, therefore, useful to ask the patient to point to the exact location where possible to eliminate a range of causes associated with abdominal pain/discomfort. For example, appendix pain may start in the central abdomen and then localise to the right lower quadrant (Welsby, 2002). Any radiation of the symptom/pain should also be noted. A patient may present with abdominal pain, when on further exploration may also radiate into the back which is suggestive of aortic aneurysm. Without asking the relevant questions to explore radiation, the true extent of the problem may never be discovered (Crumbie, 2006).

Severity

This refers to the severity of the symptom/pain has on the patient. Asking patients to compare it with previous common type presentations such as toothache, earache, menstrual cramp is of some benefit, but the use of a pain scale would offer a robust method of diagnosing or measuring the patients' pain intensity. The most commonly used scales are visual, verbal and numerical or some combination of all three forms. The practitioner must decide whether a score given is realistic within their experience – for instance, a pain score of 10 for a stubbed toe is likely to be exaggerated. The scales may also be used for assessing pain/symptom now, compared to the time of onset, or pain on movement. It may also be used to reassess pain after the administration of analgesia to assess the efficacy of their treatment. There are alternative assessment tools which can be used if a patient is unable to vocalise a score. One such method is the use of Wong–Baker FACES Pain Rating Scale (Wong and Baker, 1988). This uses cartoon faces with different expressions to assess and it is commonly used with children. Patients are often descriptive with their symptom/pain and reflect how it is affecting them rather than describing it as the health professional would interpret the problem. It is useful to record direct quotations from the patient such as 'Feels like a stabbing knife' and 'It's like being crushed'.

Timing

Patients can often overestimate the duration of the pain/symptom, so determining the timing is an important factor in several illness/injury processes (Crumbie, 2006). It is important to ask the patient how long the condition/pain has been going on and how it has changed since onset (better, worse, different symptoms); if no longer a problem/discomfort, when did it end, how long has it lasted or lasts for, the timing in the day, the pattern of the symptom, its consistency or if it is intermittent. This is also important as symptoms can change suddenly from chronic to acute; acute to life-threatening; urgent to non-urgent.

Mechanism of injury

For patients presenting with injuries, a different approach for obtaining an HPC is required. An injury is a mechanical process that can cause damage to the skin, muscles, organs and bones. Therefore, it is important to establish the mechanism of injury (MOI) to determine the extent and severity of the injury and also to anticipate any immediate or potential problems the injury may provoke. The general rule of thumb is to ask when, how, where, what, who and why. These are referred to as Kipling's six honest men, trusty questions, and we will get to the facts in every situation (Purcell, 2010). Box 1.6 illustrates some key questions using this framework.

Box 1.6   Mechanism of injury

When did this happen?	Signs and symptoms occur at different times following injuries which will indicate the severity of the injury
How did it happen?	Relate to mechanical factors – speed, direction, height, duration and any other element
What caused the injury?	Knife (type and length), broken glass, crushed by machinery?
Where did it happen?	Have they fallen on grass or concrete? Fallen down 2 steps or 16 steps?
Why did this happen?	Has the patient fallen? Do they remember falling? Ask why they fell, if unknown, consider medical reasons
Who caused the injury?	Human, animal, insect bite wound?
	Consider non-accidental injury, domestic violence

Data from Purcell (2010).

Red flags

It is vital to check for the presence or absence of red flags. Red flags are clinical features that indicate a serious condition is present and may require urgent attention. For example, when assessing patients with acute or chronic low back pain, check for the presence or absence of the red flags such as saddle anaesthesia and/or bladder dysfunction that is suggestive of cauda equina syndrome. Central crushing chest pain is a major clinical feature of a myocardial infarction but for some patients such as the elderly, people with diabetes and women, there may be a little or no chest pain.

Past medical history

Previous illnesses and surgery

Once the patient has given an account of the presenting illness/injury, a general medical history should be established (Purcell, 2010). The past medical history (PMH) can often be a significant factor to understand the presenting illness of the patient as they are often related. It is important to establish whether the patient has any known medical problems such as diabetes, asthma, chronic obstructive pulmonary disease (COPD) or coronary heart disease (CHD). Open-ended questions, for example 'do you have any medical problems?', can be too generalised as patients can often consider this as insignificant and omit this information. It may be more appropriate to ask closed questions, for example 'do you have asthma, diabetes?'. Another helpful mnemonic is *JAM THREADS* (see Box 1.7), which will identify common medical conditions, but further questions may be required.

Box 1.7   Mnemonic for obtaining past medical illnesses

J jaundice
A anaemia and other haematological conditions
M myocardial infarction
T tuberculosis
H hypertension and heart disease
R rheumatic fever
E epilepsy
A asthma and COPD
D diabetes
S stroke

Other key areas to explore are previous hospital admissions including when and why; previous surgery; recent history of foreign travel, including immunisations taken before travelling; childhood immunisations and other immunisations such as tetanus and influenza. In relation to the presenting illness, exploring risk factors are essential. For example, if a patient presents with chest pain, ask specifically about previous episodes of angina, myocardial infarction or hypertension. According to Marsh (1999), exploring the components of the PMH takes the most skill, as an awareness of the likely differential diagnosis is needed and more importantly, this is paramount for safety in treatment regimens as contraindicated treatments must be avoided.

Drug history

A list of current prescribed medications with doses is a minimum requirement. A detailed drug history (DH) is vital as it may give an indication of disease processes that the patient was either unaware of and/or fail to disclose this information. Patients can often perceive to have no medical conditions if it is controlled effectively with medication; for example, thyroxine suggestive of hypothyroidism, salbutamol suggestive of asthma, metformin suggestive of type 2 diabetes.

The patient's current medication may also be the cause of their symptoms as a result of the withdrawal of therapy, e.g. sudden withdrawal of benzodiazepines will induce seizures and adverse drug reaction (ADR) causing unwanted effects from drugs. There is a vast amount of drugs now in use, and the effect of this has led to an increase of ADRs which account for 5% of hospital admissions (Greenstein, 2004). The majority of ADRs are common, harmless and of no clinical importance. In contrast, less common adverse reactions are potentially harmful, which can be fatal. Rawlins and Thompson (1991) proposed two types of ADRs and classify these as type A and type B.

Type A ADRs are common and are due to the normal pharmacological reactions of the drug. They are dose dependant and predictable and together they cause unwanted effects after a normal or higher than normal dose (Bennett and Brown, 2003) They are readily reversible on reducing dose or withdrawing treatment. Table 1.1 provides some well-known examples of type A reactions. Conversely, type B ADRs are pharmacologically unexpected, unpredictable and not dose dependant (Greenstein, 2004). They are less common and only occur in susceptible individuals. Examples of type B ADRs include anaphylaxis with penicillin and agranulocytosis with chlorpromazine. Type B ADRs have a low incidence, but when they do occur, they tend to be more serious. Patients at increased risk from drug interactions include the elderly and those with impaired renal or liver function (Joint Formulary Committee, 2012). Furthermore, the severity of the reaction will vary from one patient to another.

Once established, a DH is important to ascertain whether or not they are, in fact, taking them and how long they have taken medication. Studies have revealed that only about a third of general practice patients take medication as prescribed (Welsby, 2002). Patients do not like to admit they have not taken their medication, and the exploration of this must be sensitively undertaken in an attempt to not appear judgemental. Reviewing the medication with the patient, taking into account the dates they were prescribed, the dosages, frequency and route will give a good indication of compliancy. Using statements such as 'do you ever forget to take your tablets?' or 'do you have difficulty taking your tablets?' or 'when was the last time you took your medication?' may give clues to whether the patient has taken their medication. Nevertheless, Marsh (1999) states that even when approached sensitively, few patients admit to poor concordance. Some

Table 1.1   Examples of common type A ADRs and their pharmacological basis

Drug(s)	ADR	Pharmacological cause
Antibiotics	Diarrhoea, *Clostridium difficile* colitis, thrush	Disruption of normal intestinal/mucosal flora
Calcium channel blockers	Headache, peripheral oedema, flushing, palpations, heart block (diltiazem and verapamil only)	Peripheral vasodilation Blocking of cardiac conduction system
Digoxin	Arrhythmias, heart block	Slowing of atrioventricular (AV) conduction
Immunosuppressant	Susceptibility to infection, increased risk of cancers	Depression of immune system
Levodopa	Hypomania, psychosis, nausea, vomiting	Action on many cerebral dopaminergic neurones
Loop diuretics	Hypokalaemia, hypernatraemia, hypomagnesaemia, increased calcium excretion, hypotension	Diuretic activity (on renal tubules), with 'unbalancing' of iron excretion
NSAIDs	Peptic ulcer, acute renal failure, exacerbation of asthma, etc.	Blockade of physiological prostaglandin synthesis
Tricyclic antidepressants	Drowsiness, dry mouth, blurred vision, constipation, urinary retention, cardiac arrhythmias	Disruption of autonomic control (antimuscarinic anticholinergic effect)

factors may lead to non-concordance with medication such as side effects, perceived lack of efficacy and ignorance. It is therefore to establish any reasons for this. In addition, clinical conditions may affect the patient's mental status such as hypoxia resulting from exacerbation of COPD or asthma or hyperpyrexia. This can lead to patients forgetting to take any medication or conversely taking a double dose. In these circumstances, it is important to see the packages to check whether the correct number has been taken since the date prescribed.

You would also need to ask specifically about the use of over-the-counter medication such as paracetamol and herbal/homeopathic health food type preparations such as vitamins. Always ask women in the appropriate age group whether they take the oral contraceptive. These are often not considered to be 'medication' and patients will not disclose this information if not prompted.

Allergies

Establishing any known allergies caused by drugs, environmental factors, foods, and wound dressings and other agents are essential as this may be the cause of their symptoms. Allergic reactions cause a number of clinical disorders such as the following:

- Acute anaphylaxis
- Serum sickness

- Rashes
- Renal disorders
- Other allergies

Penicillin and related antibiotics are the most common cause of drug allergies. Many people confuse an uncomfortable, but not serious, ADR to a drug (such as nausea). This would be categorised a type A ADR, and not type B. For example, people who experience stomach discomfort after taking aspirin (type A ADR) often say they are allergic to aspirin; however, this would not be categorised as a type B ADR (Porter et al., 2009). For that reason, it is significant to recognise the differences.

Establishing any food allergies is a necessity, as well as medication allergies. Foods such as poultry, meat and dairy products which are protein based; eggs which contain albumin; or sea food which is often rich in iodine may be highly significant as protein, iodine or albumin-based medications or vaccine may cause a serious allergic reaction. Recording the specific nature and severity of any allergies and the allergic reaction is important in any history, irrespective of a focused or comprehensive history as this is vital for the safe administration of medicines.

Family history

The patient's family medical history is significant as there is often discernible genetic component of some medical problems such as:

- Hypertension
- Coronary heart disease
- Cancer
- Type 2 diabetes mellitus
- Inflammatory bowel disease
- Mental illnesses or mental health problems

or possible inherited diseases such as inherited haemolytic anaemia more commonly in the appropriate ethnic group (Marsh, 1999), for example:

- Sickle cell anaemia – especially in Sub Saharan Africans and malarial areas
- Thalassaemia – especially in those from the Mediterranean, Middle East, India, Southeast Asia

Try to establish the current and previous health of parents. Consider asking 'Are your mother and father living?' If not, establish age and cause of death. In a similar manner, ask about any other health problems they had, as you could miss a disease with an important familial risk; for example, the father may have died of stroke but may have had lung cancer. If parents are alive, consider asking 'has anyone in your family had similar problems?' and 'do any diseases run in the family?'.

Social history

The social determinants of health are the conditions in which people are born, grow, live, work and age (World Health Organisation (WHO), 2010). Fundamentally, the social history (SH) is crucial as it provides information on how the illness/injury and the patient interact at a functional level. Assessment of the patient's appearance, manner and general conversation will provide some social background, but more specific questions may have to be asked. It may explain behaviour of the patient in relation to illness or loss. It may also give clues as to the cause of an illness/injury. For example, changes in recent lifestyle (stress at home or work, financial difficulties) may be the precipitant for angina or developing non-cardiac chest pain.

It is necessary to find out who the patient lives with, housing, employment status/education, dependants, carer responsibilities and hobbies and interests. Ascertaining the patient's functional status will direct your questioning to the abilities to perform basic ADLs such as eating, bathing and dressing. The ability to perform ADLs will reflect and affect the patient's health, and the sudden changes in ADLs are valuable diagnostic clues. If the older patient stops eating, becomes confused or incontinent, or stops getting out of bed, then you will need to find out the underlying medical problems. Keep in mind the possibility that the problem may be acute. The SH may be basic or very complex and how much information you need to obtain will depend on the individual circumstances. Smoking, alcohol consumption and the use of recreational drugs is also relevant when obtaining the SH.

Smoking

The health risks of smoking are extensive and continue for years even after the patient has given up. Recording the patient's smoking history can be a sensitive issue as some people who smoke may feel they are being judged by healthcare professionals (Crumbie, 2006). Conversely, some patients will often say they smoke less than they actually smoke. You will need to ask 'what they smoke (cigarettes, cigars, pipe etc.)', 'how many they smoke daily' and 'for how long'. This is reported as pack years and this is calculated by multiplying the number of packs of cigarettes smoked daily by the number of years of smoking. It is generally accepted that a pack contains 20 cigarettes, and Box 1.8 demonstrates how this is calculated. A pack year history of greater than 15 increases the patient's risk of long term lung disease and could be a valuable clue in the history taking. It is also important to note if a patient does not smoke. If so, have they ever smoked, how much and how long or when he or she gave up. If a patient hesitates before saying 'no', it may be because they smoke illegal substance such as cannabis and this should be explored carefully (Rushforth, 2009).

Box 1.8   Pack years

If a patient has smoked 20 a day for 12 years
1 pack (20 cigarettes) × 12 years = 12 pack year history

If a patient has smoked 40 a day for 12 years
2 pack (40 cigarettes) × 12 years = 24 pack year history

If a patient has smoked 10 a day for 30 years
$\frac{1}{2}$ pack (10 cigarettes) × 30 years = 15 pack year history

---

Alcohol and recreational drugs

The harmful use of alcohol is one of the main risk factors to health and often directly contributes to symptoms and the need for care and treatment for illnesses and injuries.

It is responsible for about 2.3 million premature deaths worldwide per year (WHO, 2009). Injuries – both unintentional and intentional – account for more than a third of the burden of disease attributed to alcohol consumption. These include injuries from road traffic crashes, burns, poisoning, falls and drowning as well as violence against oneself or others (WHO, 2009).

Health professionals hesitate to ask patients about the use of alcohol. In some incidents, the smell of alcohol is usually easily detected but heavy drinkers who have stopped drinking before seeking help often have a sweet acetaldehyde breath (Welsby, 2002). Assessment should not go on detection of smell and an attempt should be made to estimate consumption for the patient including what the patient sees as alcohol. Often, people will underestimate the amount of alcohol consumption due to embarrassment (Rushforth, 2009) or may feel they are being judged as social deviants (Crumbie, 2006). Several patients do not perceive wine and beer as alcohol (Bickley and Szilagyi, 2009), but more importantly would not consider alcohol as a drug. Alcohol can cause serious ADRs (see Drug History) and therefore should be avoided when certain drugs are taken. For example,

- *Metronidazole* interferes with the metabolism of alcohol, causing nausea, flushing, headaches and sweating
- *Hypnotics and sedatives* are potentiated by alcohol
- *Warfarin's* anticoagulant action is enhanced with an acute overdose of alcohol
- *Metformin* carries a risk of lactic acidosis with alcohol

- *Aspirin* and other *non-steroidal anti-inflammatory drugs (NSAIDs)* carry a small risk of increased risk of gastric bleeding

When ascertaining alcohol intake, try to use open-ended questions by asking the patient

'What do you like to drink?'
'How much do you drink?'
'When was your last drink?'
'Tell me about your use of alcohol?'

If you are having problems getting truthful answers or have concerns about the misuse of alcohol, ask the patient 'if they have ever had a drinking problem'. There are also validated screening tools you can use to support your assessment. The WHO (1980) developed the Alcohol Use Disorders Identification Test (AUDIT) which is a brief screening tool developed for use in primary care settings. The most widely used screening questions are about Cutting down, Annoyance if criticised, Guilty feelings and Eye-openers, (CAGE) (Ewing, 1984). When questioning, you should ask the following:

Have you ever felt the need to *cut down* on drinking?
Have you ever felt *annoyed* by criticism of your drinking?
Have you ever felt *guilty* about drinking?
Have you ever taken a drink first thing in the morning (*eye opener*) to steady
    your nerves or get rid of a hangover?

The CAGE questions should not be preceded by any questions about alcohol intake as its sensitivity is dramatically enhanced by an open-ended introduction (Steinweg and Worth, 1993). Two or more affirmative answers to the CAGE questions suggest alcohol misuse (Bickley and Szilagyi, 2009), nevertheless this cannot lead you to conclude beyond doubt that there is a problem as the diagnostic accuracy for the CAGE framework has not been fully established (Taner and Antony, 2004).

Following on from alcohol screening it would be appropriate at this point to enquire specifically about the use of recreational drugs particularly if needle marks are spotted or the patient presents with a decreased level of consciousness or possible misuse of prescription drugs. As with alcohol, the questions need to be focused if you are to get meaningful answers. Rushforth (2009) suggests that you need to ask this question sensitively as some patients will be offended whereas Welsby (2002) recommends that you ask outright, 'What drugs do you take?'. If nonusers are offended, this will be easily recognised and you can immediately respond by saying 'I mean medical drugs such as painkiller or tablets for your blood pressure'. Drug users will give a truthful answer. From this, you can establish about either patterns of use (last use, how often, substances used, amount) and/or route of administration (oral, smoking or injecting). The CAGE questions can be adapted to screen for substance abuse by adding 'or drugs' to each question.

Mental health history

One in four people will experience some kind of mental health problem in the course of a year (Office for National Statistics, 2001), and ambulance staff and ambulance crews will frequently be the first contact for many patients with mental ill health in a crisis (Department of Health (DH), 2004). Furthermore, it is estimated that up to 5% of those attending an emergency department have a primary diagnosis of mental ill health, of which substance misuse and deliberate self-harm (DSH) are the largest groups (DH, 2004); 400 per 100,000 patients in the United Kingdom will self-harm (Mental Health Organisation, 2010). A further 20–30% of attendees have co-existing physical and psychological problems, with much of the latter remaining undetected (DH, 2004). Recognition of mental health problems is essential, yet can pose challenges in any environment due to the interplay between mental disorders and physical health. Mental health disturbances can present with physical symptoms (somatisation) and/or with signs suggestive of physical illness (Welsby, 2002), and physical illness can present with behavioural and emotional responses (Bickley and Szilagyi, 2009).

Typically, the 'general medical' mental health assessment is very detailed (Welsby, 2002) and this level of detail would not be commonly undertaken in the pre-hospital setting (Gregory and Murcell, 2010), emergency and urgent care setting. The medical history would include social and physical aspects but the patient's appearance, dress and demeanour may all be important clues to the presence of a mental disorder (Welsby, 2002). It may be necessary to obtain further background information to establish low mood, anxiety and depression. This includes the following:

- Experience of childhood
- Adolescence
- Occupation(s)
- Marital history
- Previous mental health
- Problems with current life situation
- Problems with various addictions (including alcohol and drugs)

The *SAD PERSONS* risk assessment tool (see Table 1.2) will be useful when assessing the risk of DSH. Nonetheless, assessing suicide risk is very complex and as a result, there is limited evidence to support the use of this tool.

Table 1.2   SAD PERSONS assessment

Sex	Female	Male
Age	19–45	<19 >45
Depression or hopelessness	No	Yes
Previous attempts	No	Yes
Excessive alcohol or drugs	No	Yes
Rational thinking	Yes	No
Separated/divorced/widowed	No	Yes
Organised or serious attempts	No	Yes
Social support	Yes	No
Stated future suicide intent	No	Yes
		Number of ticks in this column indicates score
		<3 low risk
		3–6 medium risk
		>6 high risk

Data from Patterson et al. (1983).

Sexual health

Obtaining a sexual history is often not appropriate in the pre-hospital, emergency and urgent care environment unless it is relevant to their presenting problem such as vaginal or penile discharge or where pregnancy may be a complication such as lower abdominal pain which has the potential to be an ectopic pregnancy. A sexual history should also be considered together with a urinary history, if the patient presents with a urinary problem. Due to the close location of the urinary and reproductive systems, it can be difficult for you and the patient to differentiate signs and symptoms.

Many patients (and sometimes healthcare practitioners) are not willing to discuss their sexual history with a healthcare practitioner due to feeling embarrassed and uncomfortable (Tomlinson, 1998); consequently, it is essential to be tactful and sensitive to this. Men, particularly younger men, older people, people from different cultures and teenagers may all have particular sensitivities about the sexual health issues they need to discuss. It is important to think about the young people in particular, in respect of their age, the age of sexual partners, competency to consent, confidentiality and safeguarding.

When taking a sexual history, it is vital that you feel comfortable discussing their problem, as this will encourage the patient to talk openly. Begin with explaining to the patient for having to ask sensitive questions and why it is appropriate.

Review of systems

A history is not complete without a review of systems. The questions commonly pertain to symptoms, but can sometimes include diseases such as pneumonia or tuberculosis (Bickley and Szilagyi, 2009). The purpose of this is to search for hidden clues to uncover problems that the patient has overlooked, particularly in areas that are not related to the presenting problem; and to double check that significant information has not been left out. It is usual to start the review in a logical order from 'head to

Box 1.9	Review of systems		
Nervous	Visual problems	**Urinary**	Frequency
	Hearing problems		Pain on passing urine
	Headaches		Urinary stream
	Fits/faints/blackouts		Back pain
	Muscle weakness		Urine characteristics
	Abnormal sensations		Incontinence
Respiratory	Cough	**Genital**	Pain/discomfort/ itching
	Sputum production		
	Haemoptysis		Discharge
	Chest pain		Unusual bleeding
	Shortness of breath		Sexual history, if relevant
	Wheezing		
Cardiovascular	Chest pain	**Musculoskeletal**	Muscle weakness
	Shortness of breath		Joint swelling
	Ankle swelling		Joint pain
	Palpitations		Muscle pain
Gastrointestinal	Appetite		Cramp
	Weight change		Loss of strength
	Difficulty in swallowing		
	Pain on swallowing		
	Nausea or vomiting		
	Abdominal pain		
	Jaundice		
	Change in bowel habit		
	Heartburn, indigestion, flatulence		
	Haematemesis, melaena		

toe', and start with the general questions as you address each system. For example:

'How are your ears and hearing?'
'How are you at remembering things?'
'How about your lungs or breathing?'
'Do you have any trouble with your heart?'
'How are your eating habits?'
'How about your bowels?'

If you identify any areas of concern, a more focused exploration will be required. Box 1.9 demonstrates some key examples.

Summary

History taking is a fundamental skill in clinical practice and the importance of history taking and why we need to obtain thorough accurate data cannot be over emphasised. To achieve that requires a vast range of knowledge and skills such as communication, history-taking methods, pathophysiology, prevalence of disease, differential diagnosis to name a few, to ensure the patient receives the appropriate care and management. There are several models that can be used to guide the history taking process and depending on the situation of the clinical incident, the correct approach will be used. However, for the majority of patients the traditional medical model is the preferred method to ensure that relevant data is collated. This chapter has briefly introduced some basic methods, but has focused predominantly on the traditional medical model together with some useful mnemonics that can be used to structure your questioning.

History taking is a complex process as you need to consider other factors of relevance such as the PMH, DH and the psychosocial aspects and this chapter has explored the importance of capturing this data and its relationship to the patient's clinical condition. It is evident that communication is vital in the history-taking process and this has been briefly introduced. As a vast subject area, this has been explored fully in Chapter 2 and it is highly recommended that you read this chapter in conjunction with this to fully understand the impact, both positive and negative, this will have when obtaining information to assess and manage care effectively.

References

Bennett, P.N. & Brown, M.J. (2003) *Clinical Pharmacology*, 9th edn. Elsevier, London.

Bickley, L.S. & Szilagyi, P.G. (2009) *Bates' Guide to Physical Examination and History Taking*, 10th edn. Lippincott Williams and Wilkins, London.

Clarke, C. (1999) Taking a history. In: *Nurse Practitioners. Clinical Skills and Professional Issues* (eds M. Walsh, A. Crumbie & S. Reveley), pp. 3–13. Butterworth-Heinemann, Oxford.

Crumbie, A. (2006) Taking a history. In: *Nurse Practitioners. Clinical Skills and Professional Issues*, 2nd edn (ed. M. Walsh), pp. 14–26. Elsevier, London.

Department of Health (2004) *Improving the Management of Patients with Mental Health in Emergency Care Setting*. Department of Health, London.

Duffy, J. (1999) Therapeutic communication and the nurse practitioner. In: *Nurse Practitioners: Clinical Skills and Professional Issues* (eds M. Walsh, A. Crumbie & S. Reveley), pp. 249–259. Butterworth-Heinemann, Oxford.

Epstein, O., Perkin, G.D., Cookson, J. & de Bono, D.P. (2008) *Clinical Examination*, 4th edn. Mosby, Edinburgh.

Ewing, J.A. (1984) Detecting alcoholism: the CAGE questionnaire. *Journal of American Medical Association*, **252**(140), 1905–1907.

Gask, L. & Usherwood, T. (2002) ABC of psychological medicine. The consultation. *British Medical Journal*, **3249**(7353), 1567–1569.

Greenstein, B. (2004) *Trounce's Clinical Pharmacology for Nurses*, 17th edn. Elsevier, London.

Gregory, P. & Murcell, I. (2010) *Manual of Clinical Paramedic Procedures*. Wiley-Blackwell, Oxford.

Joint Formulary Committee (2012) *British National Formulary 64*. Pharmaceutical Press, London.

Kaufman, G. (2008) Patient assessment: effective consultation and history taking. *Nursing Standard*, **23**(4), 50–56.

Marsh, J. (1999) *History and Examination*. Mosby, London.

Mental Health Organisation (2010) http://www.mentalhealth.org.uk/infor mation/mental-health-overview/statistics/#howmany (accessed June 2011).

Morton, P.G. (1993) *Health Assessment in Nursing*, 2nd edn. F.A. Davis, Philadelphia.

Office for National Statistics (2001) Psychiatric morbidity among adults living in private household, 2000. HMSO, London.

Patterson, W.M., Dohn, H.H., Bird, J. & Patterson, G.A. (1983) Evaluation of suicidal patients: the SAD PERSONS scale. *Psychosomatics*, **24**(4), 345–349.

Porter, R.S., Kaplan, J.L. & Homeier, B.P. (2009) *The Merck Manual Home Health Handbook*. Merck Research Laboratories, New Jersey.

Purcell, D. (2010) *Minor Injuries. A Clinical Guide*, 2nd edn. Elsevier, London.

Rawlins, M.D. & Thompson, J.W. (1991) Mechanisms of adverse reactions. In: *Davies's Textbook of Adverse Drug Reactions*, 5th edn (eds D.M. Davies, R.E. Ferner & H. de Glenville). Chapman and Hall Medical, London.

Rushforth, H. (2009) *Assessment Made Incredibly Easy*, UK edn. Lippincott Williams and Wilkins, London.

Snadden, D., Laing, R., Masterton, G., Nicol, F. & Colledge, N. (2005) History taking. In: *MacCleod's Clinical Examination* (eds G. Douglas & F. Nicol), pp. 8–35. Elsevier, London.

Steinweg, D.L. & Worth, H. (1993) Alcoholism: the keys to the CAGE. *American Journal of Medicine*, **94**(5), 520–523.

Taner, M.T. & Antony, J. (2004) Reassessment of the CAGE questionnaire by ROC/Taguchi methods. *International Journal of Technology Assessment in Health Care*. **20**(2), 242–246.

Tomlinson, J. (1998) ABC of sexual health: taking a sexual history. *British Medical Journal*, **317**(7172), 1573–1576.

Welsby, P.D. (2002) *Clinical History Taking and Examination*, 2nd edn. Churchill Livingstone, London.

Wong, D.L. & Baker, C.M. (1988) Pain in children: comparison of assessment scales. *Pediatric Nursing*, **14**(1), 9–17.

World Health Organisation (1980) *Screening and brief intervention for alcohol problems in primary health care*. Available at http://www.who.int/substance_abuse/activities/sbi/en/ (accessed April 2011).

World Health Organisation (2009) *Alcohol and Injuries. Emergency Department Studies in an International Perspective*. World Health Organisation, France.

World Health Organisation (2010) *Social determinants on health*. Available at http://www.who.int/social_determinants/en/ (accessed April 2011).

2 Consultation and Communication Skills

Karen Gubbins[1] and Val Nixon[2]

[1] Institute of Health and Society, University of Worcester, Worcester, UK
[2] Faculty of Health Sciences, Staffordshire University, Stafford, UK

Introduction

Communication is a vital part of any healthcare professionals' role and is something we take for granted. When taking a medical history, effective communication is one of the best ways to obtain information from a patient; at the same time, facilitate a patient centred approach. However, for 10% of patients accessing emergency services, this approach is difficult to adopt as the needs to provide immediate clinical interventions override the need to listen to the patient.

Using a traditional medical approach of obtaining information from patients provides structure and guidance of what you should be gathering; however, this is not always easy and straightforward as you might think. There is great emphasis on gathering the data and acquiring examination skills in a consultation but less importance appears to be attached to the communication process when acquiring a patient history within a diagnostic context. Communication is a common complaint reported in healthcare and 70% of medicolegal complaints fail to gather adequate data. In addition, patients will have their own agendas based upon personal experiences; their needs and perceptions; and understanding of their illness and, therefore, we need to consider how we can use our communication skills to elicit this information.

This chapter will explore consultation/communication skills within a diagnostic framework. Firstly, the chapter gives a brief overview of the aims of the consultation and the benefits of facilitating a patient centred approach. Communication skills are vital for the success of a consultation through use of verbal and non-verbal techniques and this will be offered

Professional Practice in Paramedic, Emergency and Urgent Care, First Edition. Edited by Val Nixon.
© 2013 John Wiley & Sons, Ltd. Published 2013 by John Wiley & Sons, Ltd.

paying attention to paralinguistic cues in verbal communication. Barriers to communication are equally important and ways to circumvent them will also be included. The use of consultation frameworks will conclude using a small selection of seminal consultation models and how these can be used to guide the consultation process.

Consultation/communication skills in a diagnostic context

Patients accessing emergency care services can present with complaints that are extremely diverse, and the way doctors, nurses and paramedics elicit information from patients predominantly focusses on obtaining biomedical details. In some cases, this approach is warranted, as the urgent need to identify signs and symptoms of life-threatening illness or injury is paramount. Yet, 90% of patients accessing emergency services are not critically ill or injured but seek help and advice. In addition to seeking advice, patients may also be anxious, frightened, intoxicated, misusing drugs or have unhealthy lifestyles (Byrne and Heyman, 1997). They may have psychosocial reaction to physical disease or vice versa – physical illness such as irritable bowel syndrome, asthma, tension headache can be triggered by psychosocial factors. The effects and interpretation of illness will trigger a different response to the individual depending on their view and experiences. All these factors will have different needs and concerns and it is important to elicit these concerns within a consultation. However, it has been found that nurses working in emergency care disregard the potential for anxiety and the need for support and reassurance in patients who are not severely ill or injured (Byrne and Heyman, 1997). In addition, where communication skills of junior doctors working in emergency departments have been researched, they are found to use approaches considered to be more physician/illness orientated than patient-centred (Lloyd et al., 2000). By way of similarities of patient presentations in the pre-hospital setting, this could equally be assumed for paramedic practice.

Patients rightly expect the healthcare professional to be effective communicators, and communication failures have been cited as the commonest cause of complaint by patients. The specific areas of complaint by patients are:

- failure to gather adequate and accurate information,
- failure to provide sufficient, comprehensible information to the patient,
- failure to listen to patients' concerns on psychosocial needs,
- failure to provide mutually agreed accepted relationship.

Hargie et al. (1998).

Aims of the consultation

Historically, consultations were in the remit of medicine. Within the literature, most definitions/descriptions of consultation models and skills have, therefore, been extensively reported in the medical literature from the perspective of the doctor, predominantly within the General Practitioner (GP) practice. For non-medical professionals, the evidence that is available compares consultations with GP's and nurses and examines the outcomes of the consultation (Kinnersley et al., 2000; Shum et al., 2000; Horrocks et al., 2002) rather than the process.

Consultations, however, now take place in all professions and the evidence described in the medical literature is all relevant to all healthcare practitioners.

The aims of the consultation involve two agendas:

1. The healthcare practitioner's agenda
2. The patient's agenda

This simply means to obtain the right diagnostic information (healthcare practitioner's agenda) and to understand the patient's experience of the illness (the patient's agenda); the strength lies in integrating the two through a patient centred approach. A patient centred approach puts the patient at the heart of the interaction based on the philosophy that the patient is not a passive recipient of care. It also recognises the importance of the patient's knowledge and experience and uses it to guide the interaction (Byrne and Long, 1976). Using this approach will actively explore the patient's fears, concerns, ideas and expectations and their understanding of health and illness (Stewart, 1995). Reported benefits from this approach have been a concordance relationship through shared decision-making (Carter et al., 2003); increased patient satisfaction; increased patient adherence to planned management (whether or not that decision meets patient expectations); symptom resolution; improved emotional care (Stewart, 1995; Lewin et al., 2001); reduced anxiety, certainty and confidence that the most appropriate treatment has been chosen (Llewellyn-Thomas, 1995; Edwards and Elwyn, 1999); and improved health outcomes.

It is important to consider that whilst many patients want more information than they are given and take some part in deciding about their management of care and treatments, some patients, of course, do not wish to participate in decision-making. They would prefer to be the passive recipient and prefer the healthcare professional to decide on a single course of action and to advise them accordingly. The skill lies in achieving the correct balance for each patient.

Discussion point

I want you to consider the following scenario and consider how you would feel and respond to this scenario. You may have a similar incident that you can reflect upon. Use the questions as a guide and be honest in your answers.

You have had a busy day and you have just finished attending an incident which was very unpleasant and emotional for you and your work colleague. You have 20 minutes to go before you finish your shift and you are asked to attend a patient who has fallen off a step and injured his ankle.

How would this make you feel?
What are your thoughts en route to the scene?

When you arrive on scene, you see a male (the patient) on the floor outside his house. Before you have got out of the ambulance the patient's partner comes tapping on the window, telling you to 'get a move on'. You get out the vehicle and the patient is also shouting. He is telling you to hurry up because he is in pain and unable to move his foot. As you approach the patient, he shouts and demands that you take him to hospital for an X-ray and a tetanus injection for the graze on his left knee.

How would this make you feel now?
What are your thoughts now you are on scene?
Are they any different from your initial thoughts? If yes, how different are they?
Will this affect your relationship with the patient and his partner? If yes, how will this impact on your partnership with the patient?
Do you think their attitude will have an impact on your communication skills?
What approach will you use during your consultation?
What will the outcome be for this patient?

The success of any consultation will depend on how well the healthcare practitioner and patient communicate with each other (Toop, 1998) and some healthcare professionals are much better natural communicators than others. Communication skills in consultations are numerous and sometimes nebulous but developing them can improve the consultation. Using these skills can help us to think more effectively and explore many different ways of understanding how our patients think and behave. It is important to recognise the different channels of communication to gain a broader insight and awareness about how effective or ineffective our communication can be.

Consultation/communication skills

Communication can be considered to be the process of passing information from one person to another. There are many potential methods for these transfers which include the following:

- Verbal: talking or shouting
- Written: a letter or e-mail
- Body language: leaning against a wall or frowning
- Sign language (formal or informal): use of British Sign Language, waving goodbye or shaking a fist

Communication is a two-way process, meaning that the message has to be sent by someone and received and decoded *in the way it was intended* by someone else. Figure 2.1 clearly demonstrates how messages are effectively transmitted through verbal and written communication. A failure within this process leads to miscommunication and misunderstanding. This can result in minor and/or major omissions that have the potential to lead to catastrophic outcome for the patient and healthcare professional (see Figures 2.2 and 2.3).

There could be several reasons why failures within verbal and written communication occur. This could be any of the following:

- the sender did not send or write correctly and accurately,
- the receiver did not receive or read the message clearly – 16 was heard as 60, 60 as 66
- the word 16 was not enunciated clearly
- something interfered with the word in transit between the speaker or writer and the receiver for it to be perceived as 60, reader 60 as 66.

Many other factors can interfere with verbal transfers such as the use of a different language, different dialects or accents, a noisy environment, the

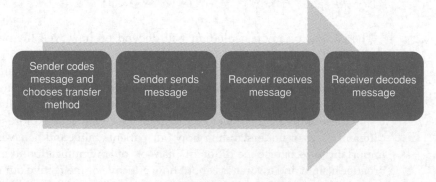

Figure 2.1   Example of how communication works.

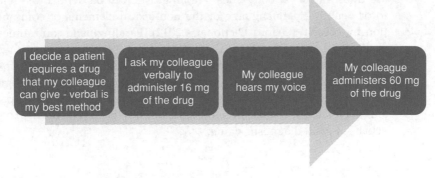

Figure 2.2   Example of verbal communication breakdown.

receiver being distracted by something else or the use of jargon. Consideration should be given to the examples given when you are using verbal and written communication, particularly, where the information being transferred is of vital importance.

Most forms of communication require considerable thought; however, because it is something we have all done for all of our lives, we take for granted that we are successful. Ask yourself how many times have you been misunderstood, or how many times have you misunderstood someone else.

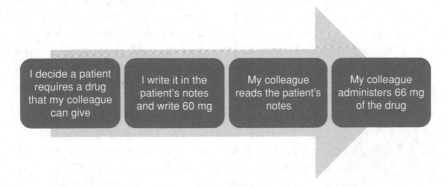

Figure 2.3   Example of written communication breakdown.

Verbal communication

Normally, when we communicate, only 7% of what we say is transmitted into words, 38% are communicated through paralinguistic cues and 55%

are transmitted via body cues. Paralinguistic can be defined as 'relating to or denoting paralanguage or the non-lexical elements of communication by speech' (Oxford Dictionary, 2012). Paralinguistic communication is therefore the verbal expression of language that does not use words, for example, the tone, pace and pitch of voice and the fluency of speech. When communicating with patients during a consultation, paralinguistic cues display a lot of meanings for the healthcare professional, the patient and the relatives. The use of paralinguistic cues that a patient displays can also be of great diagnostic value.

Pace

The pace of speech is vital to effective communication. Speaking too quickly is one of the most common speech problems – perhaps because almost all of us tend to speed up our speech when we are stressed or excited. For instance, dealing with someone who is very aggressive, attending a serious road traffic collision, being interviewed for a job, patients being anxious about their illness, worried parents – all of these situations are stressful and cause all kinds of physiological responses, including speeding up our speech. Some people, however, are genuine 'motormouths' – people who always speak rapidly. In contrast, speaking slowly is less common and people who naturally speak slowly leave gaps between words and drawls out syllables to extremes.

The speed at which you provide information could easily impact upon the amount and quality of the detail the receiver is able to decode. For instance, if you quickly bombard a patient with questions, the patient may not be able to process and decode all of the questions you have asked; therefore you may only receive one answer, or even no answer. When you speak too slowly, your listener has too much time for processing, and the mind either locks on how irritatingly slow you are speaking or wanders off to more interesting things. When talking too fast or too slow, a small part of your message will get through and most will not.

When communicating with patients, consider the speed at which they talk to you, consider using this as a guide for your speech speed. Some patient groups such as those who have cognitive difficulties; learning difficulties; who have had neurological damage caused by tumours, haemorrhagic or ischaemic stroke or trauma; the very young and the elderly may require long time to process information. However, do not assume that these groups of patients require slow speech – you need to assess the patient's abilities and adjust your communication to ensure efficacy and efficiency. Harwood (2007) examines Communication Accommodation Theory (CAT) and warns against patronising the elderly by using very simplified and slow speech. This theory could be applied to all patient groups to avoid the patient reacting negatively towards your communication attempts.

The trick to speaking at an appropriate pace is remembering that you need to speak at a rate that allows your listener to understand what you are saying. Listening is not a one-step process; we have to physically hear what is said and then translate language into meaning. If we speak too quickly, this vital second step of the process is lost.

Pitch of voice

The pitch of your voice can give different meanings to the words you say. Pitch is related to the *highness* or *lowness* of your voice. In musical terms, it is the note used; for example, the note C is different in pitch to the note A. Older patients may develop presbycusis, which is the inability to hear high-pitched sounds (National Institute on Deafness and other Communication Disorders, 2010). Therefore you may consider changing the pitch of your voice or if possible asking someone else, i.e. a colleague, to communicate verbally with the patient. Equally important is to listen to the patient's voice pitch or a child's cry for diagnostic cues. For example, a baby's cry is linked to the central nervous system and a high-pitched cry in a sick child will indicate a severe respiratory or circulatory problem.

Tone of voice

This is related to the harshness or softness of your speech and can convey a wealth of information, ranging from enthusiasm to disinterest to anger, sadness, and excitement. Consider your tone of voice when you speak to your next patient. Was it as you intended? It is easy to be quite neutral in the way we talk to patients and relatives. Think about the phrase (in a calm voice),

What can we do for you today, Mrs Smith?

How do you think Mrs Smith will respond? How would this phrase differ in context if you had shouted? Equally important is the patient's or relative's tone of voice. When a patient shouts at you, how do you respond? Do you respond by shouting back? What are the implications of doing this?

Fluency of speech

When sounds, syllables, words and phrases are joined together, speech should flow smoothly. Fluency of speech can be affected by age, gender and culture. For speech to be fluent, it needs to be understood by its speakers (speaking) and be followed and understood in the language used (comprehension). Dysfluency of speech occurs when there is an uneven flow of speech (stopping, starting, reformulating), word and sound repetitions, prolongation of sounds, etc. that interferes with communication. Fluency disorders are collectively termed as *cluttering* and *stuttering* of speech. Stuttering is a common disorder in childhood (developmental) and generally people are aware of their stuttering. Cluttering is the extreme of stuttering and affects the timing and rhythm of speech causing the person to speak too fast and as a result the speech cannot be comprehended. People who have this disorder are not aware that they are cluttering.

In terms of diagnostic value, induced fluency disorders are caused by identifiable neuropathology such as brain trauma, tumours, strokes or psychogenic which is normally triggered by an emotional crisis. Patients with mental health problems that seriously affect their thought processes and/ or language will be difficult to understand especially if it switches quickly from one unrelated idea to another (flight of ideas); or if it is long-winded and very delayed at reaching its goal (circumstantiality); or if words are inappropriately strung together resulting in gibberish (word salad).

For the remaining 55%, this is conducted through body cues that we display such as general appearance, demeanour, body language, nutritional status all of which can be open to subjectivity and assumptions and stereotypes can be formed by the receiver. During a consultation, body cues can often help you to develop appropriate communication strategies during your consultation and also support the data collected during your consultation. It is equally important to be aware of your body cues, as patients will be able see how you present yourself, sense how confident you are, and if you are calm or busy. They can also make assumptions on you as a professional and together they can all have a positive or negative impact on the consultation.

Paralinguistic communication is important to consider the reasons why they might be different and how you can adjust your communication strategies in response to this.

Non-verbal communication

A level of communication is often unconsciously motivated and may more accurately indicate a person's meaning; as opposed to the words they are being spoken. People tend to verbalise what they think a receiver wants to hear whereas less acceptable (or more honest) message may be communicated simultaneously by the non-verbal route. Non-verbal communication can encompass many things which include facial expressions, eye contact and position, body position, posture, moving of hands, touch, listening and even breathing. The use of non-verbal communication in healthcare is equally as important as verbal communication. How much do we pick up from facial expressions, general appearance, eye contact and body language?

Body language

Ford (2010) states that 'body language transcends the spoken word'. Therefore, your body language should be given a great deal of thought during a consultation. Ford (2010) goes on to suggest that our understanding of body language comes from our experiences. Therefore, cultural differences will be evident.

Much of our body language is governed by our unconscious mind, and therefore is out of our control (Boyes, 2005). However, that does not mean we cannot adapt our body language. Many aspects of body language are easy to interpret; however, it is not easy to ensure that your body language is giving the correct message. You should consider that your body displays your true feelings; therefore, if someone perceives you as disinterested, you probably are. When it comes to communicating with patients, try to remember they are individuals who deserve your full attention and actively listen to them. Active listening will ensure that you are hearing fully what they say and will show them (by your body language) that you are interested in what they have to say, thus, you are interested in them as a person. Egan (1990) suggests behaviours that form the SOLER principle.

Sit squarely opposite to the person
Open position – do not fold your arms or legs
Lean slightly towards the other person
Eye contact – maintain, but do not stare
Relax – if you are relaxed, the other person is more likely to relax

In addition, Burnard (2001) recommends prompting the other person to explain more using short sentences or questions. It can be difficult communicating with someone who displays closed manner, they may have arms and/or legs crossed and are reluctant to make or maintain eye contact. These people are displaying these signs because they may be scared or worried. Helping them to a more open body style often helps them to relax. Methods can be used to help them change to a less closed position. The first of these is to ask them to hold, pass or read something, immediately unfolding their arms. Mirroring their posture and then slowly changing your posture to a more open one can also be beneficial. Verbal communication can also assist when trying to make people more open to listening, along with assertiveness.

It is worth noting that people's body language is likely to change if they are in pain. For example, they may cradle their arm if it is injured or lean forward if they have abdominal pain.

Facial expressions

Facial expressions are movements and have the amazing ability to show a multitude of emotional expressions such as joy, surprise, fear, anger, disgust and sadness. Whilst some of these will be obvious, some can be quite subtle and open to interpretation; for example, a frown can mean you are sad, confused, angry or thinking. How does your patient or their relative know which one of these you are?

Facial expressions like any type of non-verbal communication can be very powerful and they can be out of your control at times. As with body language in general, they can communicate your true thoughts and feelings. Utilising the active listening techniques and really listening to the people talking to you will assist you in changing your expression. Also consider the facial expressions of a patient as this can also be of diagnostic value such as grimacing may indicate pain, pursing of lips – respiratory distress etc.

Facial expressions are not culturally determined but are universal across all human cultures. Facial gestures such as winking, raising an eyebrow, nodding of head indicating yes are culturally determined and it is important to be aware of the differences between facial expressions and facial gestures.

Assertiveness

Assertiveness is the ability to use language (verbal and non-verbal) to get your point across. All healthcare related situations will require some degree of assertiveness; however, the degree will depend upon the nature of the situation. Hospital experiences for many can be a frightening experience, particularly, if the patient has a serious condition. Therefore, both the patient and relative(s) will require patience and understanding. Assertiveness can assist with getting information to reluctant relatives or patients.

Assertiveness can be confused with aggression, and it can be quite easy to see how an assertive behaviour could develop into aggression. Nevertheless, when employed, appropriately assertive behaviour is far from being aggressive. It is important to consider the types of behaviours that can be considered aggressive, and those that lead to assertion. Burnard (2001) suggests examples of aggressive and assertive behaviours which are illustrated in Table 2.1.

Whilst employing these assertive behaviours, you would benefit from considering the other person's culture. Comfortable eye contact will differ from individual to individual, but what about patients who clearly do not want to make eye contact with you? Whilst you may believe you are being friendly, some cultures find eye contact acceptable and other cultures see this as unacceptable and aggressive. You need to consider how much eye

Table 2.1   Differences of assertive and aggressive behaviour

Aggressive behaviour	Assertive behaviour
Hands on hips	Face to face
Folded arms	Comfortable eye contact
Direct eye contact	Facial expression that is appropriate for the situation
Loud voice	
Threatening or angry vocal tone	Clear and calm vocal tone
Threatening or provocative gestures	

contact you are making to avoid the other person thinking you are being aggressive.

You should also consider the other person's opinions regarding the gravity of the clinical situation. As a healthcare professional, you will understand medical conditions jargon in more depth than many patients or their relatives. This can lead to complacency when explaining the medical problems to the patient. If you say, 'oh, you're just having a heart attack', think about what the patient might think and feel. It is important to remember that this patient may not have had a heart attack before, or their relatives may not have had this experience before.

Communication breakdown and barriers

There are many causes of communication breakdown which often relate to the method of communication chosen. Within the field of healthcare, Schiavo (2007) identifies nine common barriers which are as follows:

- Educational standards
- Level of healthcare knowledge
- Verbal language
- Cultural or ethical differences
- Age – young or the elderly
- Cognitive limits
- Use of jargon
- Stress related to clinical status
- Imbalance of power

It is important to adapt your communication to provide solutions to overcome these barriers and many solutions can be adopted. Some of the solutions illustrated below can be transferred to other issues and many can be used at once; therefore, they should not be considered in isolation.

Educational standard, level of healthcare knowledge and use of jargon

People come from all walks of life and; therefore, no one patient has the same knowledge as another. It is easy to use jargon and language that we are comfortable with; however, patients and relatives may not fully understand them and, therefore, what they have been told. Try wherever possible to explain in simple terms and check and clarify that the information you have passed has been understood. It is best to do this by asking the person to explain to you, in his or her own words, the information you have passed. You can then check that their understanding is correct. If you need to use jargon or you think it would be beneficial for the patient or their relative to know specific terms, it would be useful to have a glossary written or printed out for them. Some patients and their relatives could be very knowledgeable, so do not make assumptions here. General knowledge is very different to specific medical knowledge, therefore, careful questioning will help you to know what is understood. You can then provide additional information as needed. Be careful not to patronise people whilst talking in simple terms. It would be helpful to ascertain the person's knowledge level first, if possible.

Language barriers and cultural or ethical differences

Kar and Alcalay (2001) indicate that cultural competence is the ability to function within the context of a given group using their thoughts, language, behaviours, beliefs and values. In an idyllic world, all healthcare staff would be culturally competent in all cultures; however, in the diverse culture we live in, this is unlikely (Chapter 7 discusses cultural competence in more detail).

Ethics could be considered as the belief system that someone lives by and their own personal code of conduct. Cultural and ethical requirements could be exacerbated by a language barrier. For example, a person may have the belief that they should be treated by someone of the same gender. However, if they cannot communicate this to you, they may appear to be uncooperative or even aggressive.

Being able to communicate fully with individuals is vital to ensure that cultural and ethical boundaries are understood and met appropriately. Language barriers can be frequent within certain areas of healthcare and will often prevent effective communication. Many healthcare settings have access to professional interpreters, which is helpful. However, this may not always be the case in the community and pre-hospital setting. Thought should be given to how communication can be enhanced, for example, a book of phrases written in many languages, the use of the internet or translators via telephony.

Patients may have relatives who are able to translate for them; however, consideration should be given to the reliability and validity of the information transmitted and processed when using third party, particularly where children are the translators. More importantly, you should consider the professional and legal requirements such as consent and confidentiality when using third-party information.

Critical thinking

A relative (who is the translator) is asked to obtain information from his sister (the patient) as you need to administer a drug. You, as the attending healthcare professional, inform the patient (via her brother) that you need to administer the drug, and that you need some details of her past medical history, including a drug history of prescribed, over-the-counter, herbal or illegal drugs. You tell her brother that there are some potentially serious side effects of the drug and this information is essential. The patient's brother gives you the information and states that his sister fully understands and accepts the risks. Consider the following:

- *How do you know the patient understands and has consented?*
- *Does the patient want her brother to know about her medical and social history?*
- *Do you know what the patient's brother told her and what she has told him?*
- *Would you give the drug to the patient?*

What factors would prevent the patient from disclosing all the details? Could she have a medical (chronic or terminal) or mental health condition she wants to keep to herself? Could she be pregnant, take illegal drugs? Some of these difficulties are impossible to overcome.

Age

Age in itself should not be considered a barrier. However, some young and older patients will have difficulties in communication. Some of these difficulties are not confined to the older patient, for example, hearing impairment. The most common of these in the older patient is being hard of hearing or presbycusis. The National Institute on Deafness and other Communication Disorders (2010) recommends the following actions in cases of presbycusis.

- Face the person who has a hearing loss so that he or she can see your face when you speak.
- Be sure that lighting is in front of you when you speak. This allows a person with a hearing impairment to observe facial expressions, gestures, and lip and body movements that provide communication clues.
- During conversations, turn off the radio or television.
- Avoid speaking while chewing food (or gum) or covering your mouth with your hands.
- Speak slightly louder than normal, but do not shout. Shouting may distort your speech.
- Speak at your normal rate, and do not exaggerate sounds.
- Clue the person with the hearing loss about the topic of the conversation whenever possible.
- Rephrase your statement into shorter, simpler sentences if it appears you are not being understood.

In addition, consider the use of pen and paper, a patient who has a hearing impairment may prefer to use the written word for communication. You may also wish to explore the option of sign language.

Where you have a young patient with difficulty in verbalisation, images and objects are often useful. For example, showing a child the stethoscope, then putting it on yourself or a colleague. It may also be helpful to allow the child to try it out on someone else first – where appropriate.

Parents are a useful resource when dealing with children. Normally, children will trust their parent(s) to a greater extent than they will any healthcare professional. Therefore, it may help to demonstrate a technique on a parent, or even ask the parent to undertake the technique – where appropriate and under supervision. For some children, simply being held and reassured by their parents is sufficient to allow procedures to be performed.

Healthcare professionals should be open and honest with all patients; however, this is especially true for children. It is quite easy to tell them something will not hurt, when it only causes a small amount of discomfort, but this can destroy any rapport that has been built up and potentially any future rapport.

Cognitive limitations

Where a patient has learning difficulties or a degenerative condition that leads to cognitive decline, communication can be particularly difficult. Clear jargon-free explanations along with visual aids may be beneficial. Sadly, there will be some circumstances where the cognitive ability is so poor that a two-way communication is not possible. However, it is still advisable to verbally and non-verbally communicate with these individuals. Appropriate tone of voice may be sufficient to help calm a patient, even if they do not understand the words. Equally, using touch can be very reassuring (Bledsoe et al., 2007); however, some patients may not tolerate this. It is vital to ensure that touch is used in a socially acceptable manner such as touching hands or arms (Mistovitch et al., 2000). In addition, whilst this may be acceptable for most cultural groups, it may not be acceptable for some.

Patients who have any cognitive impairment should be assessed in line with the Mental Capacity Act (2005) and treated appropriately, paying attention to section 5.1.ii of the Act which refers to acting in the person's best interests. It is important to remember that some conditions that cause cognitive impairment may be temporary, such as a high fever, a transient ischaemic attack or drug intoxication. As soon as the person regains the ability to consent or refuse treatment, they have the right to do so. (Mental Capacity is discussed further in Chapter 6.)

Stress related to clinical status

Stress can be caused by many clinical and environmental factors such as the following:

- Fear of impending death
- Fear for their future health
- Fear for loved ones
- Pain
- Inability to act or move
- Loss of locus of control

Many of these factors can be out of the control of the healthcare professional. However, clear, assertive communication could help the patient to understand their situation and to help allay their fears. Often, allowing a patient to talk about their fears can be helpful, as can allowing their relative(s) to be around them. This gives the patient an element of control and also a person they know, which can be comforting. However, some patients may prefer to be alone at times of great stress. Clear communication and respecting the patient's wishes will often help alleviate some of their stresses. It is natural for patients to be anxious regarding their condition and care, and healthcare professionals can help relieve some of this stress using clear and full explanations.

Stress caused by pain is something that can often be remedied. It is generally accepted that pain is a subjective experience, therefore, the patient should be asked and they should be treated as per their pain score. Some patients may prefer to 'tolerate' their pain; gentle advice and reassurance of the benefits of pain relief may be appropriate.

Power imbalance

> **Critical thinking**
>
> Have you ever attended a patient who was prescribed medication and on questioning they do not know what it is for? Consider the following:
>
> - *How can this patient manage their condition effectively if they do not know what it is?*
> - *Does the patient take the medication regularly?*
> - *Does the patient understand the consequences of non-compliance with their medication?*
> - *What impact could this have on their current and future health?*

Some patients and their relatives believe that the healthcare professional knows best and they will accept anything they are told without question. This can lead to a situation where the patients and relatives are given little information about their condition and possibly their management. The situation becomes one of subservience, where the patient has no power and the healthcare professional has all of the power. This can be a destructive relationship, as the patient may feel they cannot question their care and has to blindly follow the regime given. Other patients may rebel against the healthcare advice and become non-compliant. Both of these situations are poor for long term management. In the first situation, the patient is not proactive, does not seek help, does not offer new information and waits to be told what to do next. The second situation sees the patient being resistant to any new information and management choosing their path, which could be severely detrimental to their condition.

The most productive relationship is where the healthcare professional is approachable, gives appropriate clear information and is able to ask and answer questions freely. The patient needs to believe that the healthcare professional sees them as a valuable person, not a condition. This along with good communication will allow the patient some control of their condition and its management. In turn, this will empower the patient to take more of an interest, and therefore be more proactive.

Imbalance of power

Power imbalance can be remedied by asking the patient and their relatives questions about their care. By asking questions, it can become clear whether they understand their condition and whether there is a lack of knowledge. This knowledge deficit can then be addressed. Providing knowledge should be done in terms and language the patient will understand. It may be beneficial to address more serious aspects first and less serious ones at a separate time to avoid information overload. Encouraging the patient and relative(s) to ask questions about their condition and management is a good way to equal the power with the patients.

Other barriers to communication

There are a number of barriers not directly mentioned by Schiavo (2007), for example, noise and poor handwriting. A noisy environment is not always something that you can change; however, this does not remove the fact that you still need to communicate with people.

When utilising verbal communication in a noisy environment, it is beneficial to support this with something else, for example, a written note. This may be particularly important where drugs are being administered as shown in Figure 2.3. Had the receiver of the message had a written confirmation of the dose, the patient would have received the correct amount. Patient notes are therefore a vital communication tool.

Handwriting that cannot be read is as ineffective as words that cannot be understood. Individuals who have poor handwriting may be assisting others by writing in capital letters, as they tend to be clearer and more legible than cursive writing (hence, many forms require information to be written in capitals). Use of capital letters does tend to slow the writer down until such time as they are proficient; however, the slowing down of writing often makes the text more legible. Capitalisation can therefore assist in written communication.

Communication/consultation models

Within the medical literature, consultation models and communication skills models are words that are used interchangeably to describe the process that is used when gaining a medical history. Consultation models are established lists of questions or areas to be explored, and provide a framework for a consultation. They can be useful, especially to those of us who like to think and learn in a structured or organised way, especially when developing a skill such as consulting with patients.

Over the past 30 years, there have been a number of consultation models that have been described as task-orientated, skills-based, based on the provider–patient relationship or the patient's perspective of illness. Many models now incorporate more than one model to integrate both the doctor's and the patient's perspective. This includes the following:

1. The medical model – the history of the problem and the diagnosis.
2. The patient's agenda – his or her experience of the illness and injury.

There is no suggestion that any one model is better than another, they are all valid and useful in their different ways. There is duplication between them, after all they are models based on the same fundamental activity, but with different emphasis related to their origins. Models are not intended to direct the healthcare practitioner to move rigidly through the model from beginning to end, but to select and use a part of any model and as skills develop can weave components of two or more models into the same consultation.

Transactional analysis model

One of the earliest models was the transactional analysis (TA) model, which was introduced by Eric Berne in 1964 and many doctors will be familiar with this model. Berne (1964) used concepts from psychoanalysis to describe the roles that people adopt in relationships and encounters and proposed that effective communication relies on the people involved having matching ego states. The ego states are that of a child, adult and parent and are determined by the way we think, feel, behave, react and have attitudes as if we were a critical or caring parent, a logical adult, or a spontaneous or dependent child (Berne, 1964). Table 2.2 illustrated the description and behaviours of the ego states. Individuals can switch between the ego states depending upon the situation, mood, wellness and external influences. These feelings not only influence our physical activity but also influence our communication – both verbal and non-verbal. Donnelly and Neville (2008) suggest that certain words/phrases are used by someone in each of the ego state (see example in Table 2.3). Berne (1964) goes on

Table 2.2   Transactional analysis model. Description of ego states

	Child	Adult	Parental
Description	The 'inner child'. It incorporates behaviours that are similar to those displayed by the individual when they were a child	One of autonomy, decision-making and objectivity. This ego state is developed by the individual as they gain experiences and grow through life	Developed from the individual's experience of the parent figure. It incorporates the values and behaviours associated with parenting and has critical tendencies
Behaviours	Folded arms, refusing to make contact, temper tantrums, looking sad, giggling, extreme shouting, screaming or whining and pathetic	Many and varied	Soft voices tone Caring and soft Loud and authoritative Smiles, frowns, folded arms, pointing, raising eyebrows, and open arms

Data from Berne (1964).

Table 2.3   Transactional analysis model: Ego states and associated words

Ego state	Child	Adult	Parental
Associated words	I can't I won't Now Never	How? When? Who? Why? That's a possibility? Maybe we can try that	You mustn't You ought to Just get on Don't do that

Data from Donnelly and Neville (2008).

to discuss complementary ego states and identifies where the ego states complement each other to ensure effective communication is most effective (see Figure 2.4).

Many general practice consultations are conducted between a parental doctor and a child-like patient. This transaction is not always in the best interest of either party, and familiarity with the TA introduces a welcome flexibility, which can break out of the repetitious cycles of behaviour into which some consultations can degencrate (Neighbour, 2005). These actions are the ones that often we are not aware of; however, they can profoundly influence how effective communication with patients and their relatives can be. Problems in communication are more likely to occur when the people involved in the communication are using crossed transactions. It is therefore, as a healthcare professional, important to consider that first communication is at the start of the consultation.

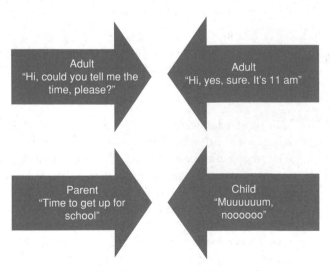

Figure 2.4   Example of effective communciation using complementary ego states.

Critical thinking

Imagine you are called out to a patient who complains of nausea. When you arrive, you initiate a conversation in the parental ego with a phrase that could be critical:

Healthcare professional: 'Why haven't you taken your medication?'
Patient: Likely to reply, but avoid eye contact, fold their arms, or even reply with a phrase like 'because I don't like it'.

What ego state is seen in the examples below?
Could this be a possible reason the patient has called you?
What impact will this have on the consultation process?
Consider the difference in an 'adult to adult' conversation:

Healthcare professional: 'Is there a problem with taking your medica-
tion?'
Patient: 'I don't like this new tablet; it makes me feel sick all of the time.'

What impact will this have on the consultation style?
Is there a potential to share decision-making, to achieve shared management and to agree for the patient to become compliant with the medication?

Body language is easily affected by the ego states, and care should be taken to prevent inappropriate messages being displayed. Consider the following examples and what ego states are likely to be displayed and what message is being sent to the patient?

A paramedic arriving at a patient's home with their hands in their pockets. A nurse on a ward is asked by a service user if she could have some water. The nurse throws her hands in the air and storms off.

In most healthcare related scenarios, it is advisable to have 'adult to adult' conversations. Patients who are older children can often respond well to an adult conversation. The utilisation of 'adult to adult' conversation allows for a good exploration of the patient's position. It ensures that they are not patronised and is, therefore, more likely to comply with requests for information or action.

Byrne and Long (1976) has another earlier model that uses six phases to form a logical structure to the consultation (see Box 2.1). The model is useful for analysing 'dysfunctional' consultations where the patient may be misunderstood and dissatisfied, while the doctor may be frustrated (Byrne and Long, 1976). It is criticised for being a heavily doctor dominated consultation through the use of direct closed questions. The patient's ideas are rejected and the doctor evades the patient's questions, and thus the patient's contribution is virtually excluded. Can you think of incidents when this model could be used?

Box 2.1	Byrne and Long – Six phase model
Phase I	The doctor establishes a relationship with the patient.
Phase II	The doctor either attempts to discover or actually discovers the reason for the patient's attendance.
Phase III	The doctor conducts a verbal or physical examination or both.
Phase IV	The doctor, or the doctor and the patient, or the patient (in that order of probability consider the condition).
Phase V	The doctor, and occasionally the patient, detail further treatment or further investigation.
Phase VI	The consultation is terminated usually by the doctor.

Data from Byrne and Long (1976).

Pendleton et al. seven task model

Pendleton et al. (1984) model is a task-orientated model and describes seven tasks which taken together form comprehensive and coherent aims for any consultation (see Box 2.2). These seven tasks are derived from joint perspectives and include the patient's needs, thoughts, ideas, anxieties and expectations, the doctor's aims, the shared desired outcomes and the linking evidence. This allows the patient to feel part of a collaborative process and to build on a practitioner–patient relationship for the future. As a comprehensive model, this may be useful for assessing and managing a patient with long term conditions as it includes the personal and psychological aspects of their illness, self-management and patient empowerment through adopting a collaborative approach.

Box 2.2   Pendleton's et al. Seven Tasks

1. To define the reason for the patient's attendance including
    I.   the nature and history of the problems
    II. their aetiology
    III. the patient's ideas, concerns and expectations
    IV. the effects of the problems

2. To consider other problems
    I.   continuing problems
    II. at-risk factors
3. With the patient, to choose an appropriate action for each problem
4. To achieve a shared understanding of the problem with the patient
5. To involve the patient in the management and encourage him to accept appropriate responsibility
6. To use time and resources appropriately
    I.   in the consultation
    II. in the long term
7. To establish a relationship with the patient which helps to achieve the other task

Data from Pendleton et al. (1984).

Neighbour's five checkpoint model

Neighbour's model (1987) is a combination of various models including Byrne and Long (1976), and Pendleton et al. tasks (1984). Neighbour (1987) describes the consultation as a journey with five 'checkpoints' along the way. These are the following:

1. Connecting
2. Summarising
3. Handing over
4. Safety netting
5. Housekeeping

This model is different from all the previous ones because it seems to have moved on to include not only the clinical components of the previous models but also now includes, for the first time, specific areas for safe doctoring (i.e. Safety Netting) and for being a healthy doctor (Housekeeping).

Connecting is established as an effective working relationship with a patient and obtaining information, developing empathy and rapport.

Summarising includes taking a history, drawing together the information gathered, making a diagnosis and summarising the problem and reflecting it back to the patient to ensure there are no misunderstandings.

Handing over is returning the responsibility for some aspects of the disease and its management to the patient. By this time, the practitioner will have brought the consultation to a point where the patient and the practitioner's agendas have been agreed on its management. This may include a range of management plans such as taking prescribed or over-the-counter medication, transporting to ED, accessing alternative pathway such as primary care services, or leaving the patient at home.

Safety netting is creating a contingency plan and procedures relevant to that patient, to ensure that the plan works out and that the patient is safe in any foreseen or unforeseen eventualities. For example, a patient who has had a hypoglycaemic attack as a result of not eating breakfast could be advised to eat carbohydrates and monitor their blood sugars and call for an ambulance or return to ED, should their blood sugars continues to fall.

Housekeeping is taking care of oneself to manage the stresses of everyday clinical practice to be at one's most efficient and effective. It recognises the need to attend to fatigue, boredom, stress, lack of concentration, distraction and all the powerful emotions that can be distracting. It may involve having a brief chat with a colleague, peer support, clinical supervision etc.

Calgary-Cambridge model

The Calgary-Cambridge approach was developed as a teaching tool for consultation skills by Kurtz and Silverman in 1996. In 2002, this was extended and developed and now offers a comprehensive guide to healthcare practitioners. This model places the disease-illness model at the centre of gathering information. It combines the process with content in a logical schema. It is comprehensive and applicable to all medical interviews with patients, whatever the context. It also reflects the changes in the later consultation models (Pendleton and Neighbour) with increasing emphasis on a patient centred consultation using five tasks:

1. Initiating the session
2. Gathering information
3. Building the relationship
4. Explanation and planning
5. Closing the session

The model also provides a framework of skills, which provide further details of the steps to be achieved within each consultation (see Box 2.3).

Box 2.3   Calgary-Cambridge Model

Initiating the session

Preparation

Establishing initial rapport

Identifying the reason(s) for the consultation which includes the bio-medical perspective and the patient perspective

Gathering information

Exploration of the patient's problems to discover the:

Biomedical perspective – the patient's perspective

Background information – context

Physical examination

Explanation and planning

Providing the correct amount and type of information

Aiding accurate recall and understanding

Achieving a shared understanding incorporating the patient's illness and framework

Planning shared decision-making

Closing the session

Ensuring appropriate point of closure

Forward planning

Data from Kurtz et al. (2003).

Discussion point

Out of the consultation models listed above, which model seems the most natural to your style of consultation?
Which one is the least natural to your style of consultation?
Which model have you predominately used in practice?
Does this differ from your most natural style?
Would you use the same model or would your style change depending on the situation?

Summary

As a healthcare professional, one of your greatest tools is communication. Communication is a complex two-way process that requires constant evaluation to ensure effectiveness to achieve the appropriate outcomes for patient and relatives that we come into contact with.

Within a diagnostic context, effective communication skills and the manner in which we use our communication skills is fundamental to achieving a patient centred approach. Developing a patient centred approach requires the healthcare practitioner to adopt a consultation style that is relaxed, open and responsive to patient cues. Utilising patient centred techniques enables us to understand what is important and concerning to the patient, it is intrinsically therapeutic and sets the consultation within a truly holistic framework. An awareness of how we communicate and how the patient communicates is fundamental to this process as communication techniques may need to be adapted and changed based on individuals. This chapter has intended to provide you with the underpinning theory of communication and how communication/consultation can be used to provide structure to your consultation to ensure a patient centred approach. We hope this has given you with some thoughts to your communication style, and ideas and techniques on how to adapt to every situation you are faced with.

References

Berne, E. (1964) *The Games People Play: The Psychology of Human Relationships.* Penguin Books, London.

Bledsoe, B., Porter, R. & Cherry, R. (2007) *Essentials of Ambulance Clinician Care,* 2nd edn. Prentice-Hall, New Jersey.

Boyes, C. (2005) *Need to Know Body Language the Secret Language of Gestures and Postures Revealed.* Collins, London.

Burnard, P. (2001) *Effective Communication Skills for Health Professionals.* Nelson Thornes, Cheltenham.

Byrne, G. & Heyman, R. (1997) Understanding nurses' communication with patients in accident and emergency departments using a symbolic interactionist perspective. *Journal of Advanced Nursing,* **26**(1), 93–100.

Byrne, P. & Long, B. (1976) *Doctors Talking to Patients.* HMSO, London.

Carter, S., Taylor, D. & Levenson, R. (2003) From compliance to concordance: a preliminary review. Available from http://www.medicines-partnership. org/research-evidence/major-reviews/a-question-of-choice (accessed June 2012).

Donnelly, E. & Neville, L. (2008) *Communication and Interpersonal Skills.* Reflect Press, Devon.

Edwards, A.G.K. & Elwyn, G.J. (1999) How should effectiveness of risk communication to aid patients' decisions be judged? A review of the literature. *Medical Decision Making,* **19**(4), 428–434.

Egan, G. (1990) *The Skilled Helper,* 4th edn. Brooks/Cole Pacific Grove, California.

Ford, M. (2010) *Body Language and Behavioural Profiling.* AuthorHouse, Bloomington, IA.

Hargie, O., Dickson, D., Boohan, M. & Hughes, K. (1998) A survey of communication skills training in UK schools of medicine: present practices and prospective proposals. *Medical Education,* **32**(1), 25–34.

Harwood, J. (2007) *Understanding Communication and Aging.* Sage, London.

Horrocks, S., Anderson, E. & Salisbury, C. (2002) Systematic review of whether nurse practitioners working in primary care can provide equivalent care to doctors. *British Medical Journal*, **324**(7341), 819–823.

Kar, S. & Alcalay, R. (eds) (2001) *Health Communication: A Multicultural Perspective.* Sage, London.

Kinnersley, P., Anderson, E., Parry, K., et al. (2000) Randomised controlled trial of nurse practitioner versus general practitioner care for patients requesting "same day" consultations in primary care. *British Medical Journal*, **320**(7241), 1043–1048.

Kurtz, S. & Silverman, J. (1996) The Calgary-Cambridge Referenced Observation Guides: an aid to defining the curriculum and organizing the teaching in communication training programmes. *Medical Education*, **30**(2), 83–89.

Kurtz, S., Silverman, J., Benson, J. & Draper, J. (2003) Marrying content and process in clinical method teaching: enhancing the Calgary-Cambridge guides. *Academic Medicine*, **78**(8), 802–809.

Lewin, S.A., Skea, Z.C., Entwistle, V., Zwarenstein, M. & Dick, J. (2001) Interventions for providers to promote a patient-centred approach to a clinical consultation. *Cochrane Database of Systematic Reviews*, (4), CD003267. doi: 10.1002/14651858.

Llewellyn-Thomas, H.A. (1995) Patients' health-care decision making: a framework for descriptive and experimental investigations. *Medical Decision Making*, **15**(2), 101–106.

Lloyd, G., Skarratts, D., Robinson, N. & Reid, C. (2000) Communication skills training for emergency department senior house officers – a qualitative study. *Journal of Accident and Emergency Medicine*, **17**(4), 246–250.

Mental Capacity Act (2005) *Mental Capacity Act (c.9.).* HMSO, London.

Mistovitch, J., Hafen, B. & Karren, K. (eds) (2000) *Pre-Hospital Emergency Care.* Prentice-Hall. New Jersey.

National Institute on Deafness and other Communication Disorders (2010) *Presbycusis.* Available at http://www.nidcd.nih.gov/health/hearing/pages/presbycusis.aspx (accessed 24, February 2012).

Neighbour, R. (1987) *The Inner Consultation. How to Develop an Effective and Intuitive Consulting Style.* Kluwer Academic Publisher, Lancaster.

Neighbour, R. (2005) *The Inner Consultation. How to Develop an Effective and Intuitive Consulting Style*, 2nd edn. Radcliffe Publishing, Oxford.

Oxford Dictionary (2012) *Definition of Paralinguistic* [online]. Available at http://oxforddictionaries.com/definition/paralinguistic?q=paralinguistic (accessed 24 February 2012).

Pendleton, D., Schofield, T., Tate, P. & Havelock, P. (1984) *The consultation: an approach to leaning and teaching.* Oxford University Press, Oxford.

Schiavo, R. (2007) *Health Communication: From Theory to Practice.* Jossey-Bass, San Francisco.

Shum, C., Humphreys, A., Wheeler, D., Cochrane, M.A., Skoda, S. & Clement, S. (2000) Nurse management of patients with minor illnesses in general practice: multicentre, randomised controlled trial. *British Medical Journal*, **320**(7241), 1038–1043.

Stewart, M.A. (1995) Effective physician-patient communication and health outcomes: a review. *Canadian Medical Association Journal*, **152**(9), 1423–1433.

Toop, L. (1998) Primary care: core values. Patient-centred primary care. *British Medical Journal*, **316**(7148), 1882–1883.

3 Clinical Decision Making

Jacqui Mason and Val Nixon

Faculty of Health Sciences, Staffordshire University, Stafford, UK

Introduction

Clinical decisions are central to healthcare practice. Paramedics are on a day to day basis responsible for the decisions around treatment and transfer of patients in the pre-hospital setting. Paramedics need to make decisions that will have a major impact on their patient's clinical outcome and safety. These decisions are based on a variety of sources of information (Thompson and Dowding, 2009) such as experience, knowledge, expertise of others, research and available evidence.

Underpinning how these decisions are made are a number of theories and models, which explain how the diversity of information available is used within the decision-making strategies that support practice. However, paramedics often have limited resources available to them in some situations, including partial or incomplete patient histories and/or limited support available from colleagues (Jensen et al., 2009). Combined with this, many pre-hospital emergency patients have high acuity and time critical conditions. Furthermore, for a variety of reasons, the information that we draw upon may, at times, be distorted or limited.

When seeking professional guidance or support other individuals that we may draw on may not have the expertise we attribute to them or the research or evidence on which we base our decisions may even be flawed. As a result, it is therefore essential to learn more about clinical decision making and apply the required skills to be justifying actions taken in clinical practice.

There is little evidence of clinical decision-making theories and frameworks and their application in paramedic practice. In addition, there is very limited empirical evidence on how exactly paramedics make decisions and, therefore, this chapter will draw from similar practice disciplines and

Professional Practice in Paramedic, Emergency and Urgent Care, First Edition. Edited by Val Nixon.
© 2013 John Wiley & Sons, Ltd. Published 2013 by John Wiley & Sons, Ltd.

health professions. The literature available in relation to theories, frameworks and methods used to offer guidance and structure to clinical decision making is often blurred as many authors offer different interpretations and evaluations of the concepts and its application.

This chapter will, therefore, provide you with an introduction to these concepts to allow you, as a paramedic, to understand the fundamentals of this vast subject area and hopefully avoid some of the pitfalls that are inevitable when making decisions. This expanded knowledge on how you make decisions will then assist you to continue to provide safe and effective decision making in the clinical area.

A brief introduction to decision making theories

The subject of how paramedics make decisions is largely unexplored; however, the subject of decision making has been studied by many authors over the last half a century (Thompson and Dowding, 2009), and each offers different terminology to describe the same phenomena. These include clinical decision making (Field, 1987; Ford et al., 1979; Luker and Kendrick, 1992); clinical judgement (Benner and Tanner, 1987); clinical inference (Hammond, 1964); clinical reasoning (Grobe et al., 1988); diagnostic reasoning (Carnevelli et al., 1984; Radwin, 1990) and judgements and decisions (Thompson and Dowding, 2009). These studies may not purely relate to the pre-hospital and paramedic practice; however, these are applicable to any clinical profession and the principles, therefore, are transferable.

To begin your understanding of the subject, it may be useful to consider a definition of clinical decision making. Goleman (2002) has stated that decision making is a case of 'choosing between different alternatives'. This seems a simple definition, and may be oversimplified, considering the complexity of decisions made in clinical practice. However, it indicates that the key aspect of a decision is the need to commit to one course of action in preference to another. This choice may be irreversible; for example, once you have cannulated a patient and made the decision to administer a drug, once administered you cannot go back on your decision and remove the drug. Standing (2010) and Tanner et al. (1987) discuss clinical decision making as a complex process, which involves many elements such as observation, information collection, information processing, recognising problems, problem recognising skills, problem solving skills, reflection and judgement. This definition can also be expanded to include consideration of ethics and professional accountability (Standing, 2010).

Ultimately, as a clinician, you will want to make good clinical decisions. Whilst the actual doing of decision making is fundamentally the most important aspect to all clinicians, by having a clear understanding and knowledge base of the theories and models of decision making you can hopefully make more informed and improved decisions. The practical examples given and explored within this chapter rely on the theoretical models of the way in which decisions are made.

Decision-making theories

Decision making tends to fall within three different theories: normative, descriptive or prescriptive; however, in reality, the distinction is rather blurred.

Normative theories are concerned with the analysis of individual decisions and are concerned with formal logic and rationality (Kahneman and Tversky, 2000). As a theory, it is concerned with identifying the optimal decision to be taken, assuming an ideal decision maker is fully informed and able to understand all areas of the decision-making process fully, accurately and rationally. In essence, the normative theories identify how someone should make a decision and behave.

Descriptive theory looks at how people make decisions in real life, how they choose between the options available to them. This theory was identified from empirical experiments, where it was shown that people's behaviour is inconsistent with normative theories.

Prescriptive decision making is a combination of the theoretical aspect of normative theory and the observations of descriptive theory. It aims to provide practical aid with decision making, whilst aspiring to rationality. Prescriptive decision theory provides a set of rules, combining belief and preferences in order to select an option, exploiting the logical consequences of normative theories and the empirical findings of a descriptive theory. Criticism that has been associated with this is that the theory may be unrealistic and may affect consistency, which is often sought after when making decisions, and can be impacted further by the sources of uncertainty that are often associated with decision making. The prescriptive theory of decision making is even more complex when decision makers have to interact with others who may think along different paradigms.

- Normative – what theory dictates people should do when making a decision
- Descriptive – what people actually do or have done when making a decision
- Prescriptive – what people should and can do when making a decision

Decision-making models

Regardless of the theories, there are many models that have been identified and used with decision making. The next section of this chapter will explore a number of these models which you may be able to relate to clinical practice.

Decision making is such a common activity that you probably rarely devote any thought to discovering what a decision is. When attempting to describe decisions and decision making, the starting point should be some form of conceptual framework or model. However, there are numerous frameworks and models used to interpret and explain the process of clinical decision making, and the diversity of explanations and the complexity of them have often masked common themes between them. Two keys opposing conceptual framework that underpin the decision-making process are the *analytical framework* (also known as deductive framework) and the *intuitive* framework (also known as inductive framework (Hamm, 1988). Inductive frameworks are where data is collected and leads to generation of a hypothesis. In contrast, deductive frameworks are when hypotheses are used to predict the presence or absence of data which clinicians then search to confirm or deny the hypotheses.

For most patient presentations, a combination of analytical and intuitive frameworks will be adopted using intuition, pattern recognition and the hypothetico-deductive approaches to clinical reasoning. These are the three commonly used approaches and will apply to everyday clinical decision making when deciding on the best course of action for the patient. However, in complex incidents such as major medical incidents, this may require a broader approach and these methods will not be appropriate to use.

Intuitive framework – heuristics approach

Intuition and pattern recognition are two main approaches within the intuitive framework.

Intuition

Intuition is simply defined as 'understanding without rationale' (Benner and Tanner, 1987) and is regarded as an alternative explanation for how we make decisions. In some situations, experts in practice can have intuitive thoughts – 'hunches', 'ideas' – of a patient's diagnosis or condition by certain words and phrases that patients use, their appearance and/or body language. Benner's (1984) infamous work identified five stages of skills acquisition and development (see Table 3.1) and found that judgements of experts were different from those of with less expertise. Novices rely on analytical principle to understand the current situation and to guide their actions whereas the expert no longer relies on analytical principles but uses intuition instead.

Table 3.1   Benner's 5 stage acquisition model

Stage	Brief description
1. Novice	Beginners have no experience of the situation on which to draw and rules and regulations are extremely limited and inflexible.
2. Advanced beginner	Unlike principles and rules, aspects of overall characteristics of a situation that can only be identified from experience. Can demonstrate marginally acceptable performance gained from sufficient prior experience. Able to discriminate between normal and abnormal findings but not able to focus on advanced skills of judging the relative importance of different aspects of the situation that may result in abnormal findings.
3. Competent	Conscious deliberate planning based upon analysis and careful deliberation of situations. Able to identify priorities and manage their work. Learning activities will be the centre of decision making, for example, the competent professional when interviewing patients will be able to obtain subjective data and also consciously observe a patient's physical and psychosocial behaviour. This will allow overall analysis to determine priorities to deliver effective responsive care.
4. Proficient	Is able to perceive situations holistically and at this stage the keyword is perception. The perception is not thoughout but 'present itself' based on experience and recent events. Has the ability to recognise the whole situation. Holistic understanding improves clinical decision making and it becomes less laboured as they are able to consider fewer options and focus directly on the most relevant aspects of a problem.
5. Expert	Expert performers have a huge wealth of experience and no longer rely on analytical principles to connect their understanding of the situation. This stage is characterised by a deep understanding and an intuitive grasp of the total situation. Expert, intuitive clinicians cannot always give a rational for their actions. Expert clinicians are not difficult to recognise because they frequently make clinical judgments or manage complex clinical situations in a truly remarkable way.

Data from Benner (1984).

Experts in practice tend to have an intuitive grasp of each situation and focus on the direct problem without wasteful considerations of a large range of unnecessary, alternative diagnosis and solutions. For instance, for a patient who complains of severe back pain who is pale and clammy, an expert paramedic would immediately consider a ruptured abdominal aneurysm. Benner (1984) supports this and argues that intuition is an essential part of clinical judgement and is linked clearly to the expertise. Capturing descriptions of expert performance though is difficult because it is characterised by having a deep understanding and intuitive grasp of the total situation. Critics would argue that it is purely guesswork, based on personal opinion. Consequently, the evidence for the use of intuition is anecdotal, and the inability of defining and quantifying this phenomenon has been contributed by the feeling that it is unreliable, unscientific and somehow unworthy. In an attempt to understand intuition, Carper (1978) identified four ways of knowing. The typology identifies four fundamental 'patterns of knowing':

1. *Empirical:* Factual knowledge from science, or other external sources, that can be empirically verified.

2. *Personal:* Knowledge and attitudes derived from personal self-understanding and empathy, including imagining one's self in the patient's position.
3. *Ethical:* Attitudes and knowledge derived from an ethical framework, including an awareness of moral questions and choices.
4. *Aesthetic:* Awareness of the immediate situation, seated in immediate practical action; including awareness of the patient and their circumstances as uniquely individual, and of the combined wholeness of the situation.

Intuition is an escapable part of clinical decision making and should not be ignored. If your gut feeling is telling you there is something wrong, then it most probably is. You should not ignore your feelings and continue to assess the patient to support your initial thoughts. You can often find subtle findings based on the patient's appearance, their demeanour or words spoken by the patient and you should continue looking to support this.

> **Discussion point**
>
> How often have you known that a patient was critically ill, when you are unable to obtain factual information to support your feeling?
> How often have your thoughts been proven to be accurate?
> What evidence have you collated to prove this?
> What is your explanation of this?

Pattern recognition

Pattern recognition is a popular term for describing decision making (Benner et al., 1996). This approach is usually cited in connection with intuition as a pattern of cues will generate outcomes without conscious awareness of the process and equally uses terms such as 'gut feeling', salience, gestalt and hunch. (Buckingham and Adams, 2000). When using pattern recognition, the practitioner uses experience and knowledge of illness and disease to recognise a pattern of symptoms or phrases used by the patient that would strongly suggest a diagnosis. For example, tight central chest pain would strongly suggest myocardial infarction; Achilles tendon rupture – patients would describe the injury as being shot in the leg (at the site of injury); thunderclap headache is suggestive of subarachnoid headache – patients would describe this as the worst headache they have ever had.

This may be the primary method used in cases where diseases are 'obvious', or the patient's previous experiences may enable him/her to recognise their condition quickly. Theoretically, a certain pattern of signs or symptoms can be directly associated with a certain therapy (e.g. cardiac chest pain), even without a definite decision regarding what is the actual disease, but such a compromise carries a substantial risk of missing a diagnosis which actually has a different therapy so it may be limited to cases where no diagnosis can be made.

> ### Discusson point
>
> Can you identify examples of when you have used pattern recognition?
> Have you always been accurate in your initial working diagnosis?
> Consider when this method would be appropriate to use?
> What are the implications of using this method, for you as a professional, and the patient?

Cioffi (1997) and Buckingham and Adams (2000) offer an alternative approach to explain and understand intuition, and use the term 'heuristics'. Tversky and Kahnemann (1974) have suggested that heuristics are methods of simplifying complicated decisions by using psychological shortcuts or 'rules of thumb'. Shortcuts speed up the process of finding a satisfactory solution as the shortcuts created are picked up from certain cues identified from a huge amount of information Cioffi, 1997. Based on the shortcuts, heuristics has a tendency to make probability judgements based on the similarity of an event to an underlying basis. The greater the similarity, the higher the probability estimate to the same situation will be. Although decisions made using heuristics are easy decisions to make, from a psychological point of view, they may lead to biases or irrelevant information may not be taken into account when making the decision. In reality, when making decisions, we often 'satisfice'; whereby we select the option that meets acceptable standards as an efficient form of decision making. This concept has been expanded on by Gigerenzer and Todd (1999) to apply 'fast and frugal' heuristics that take advantage of environmental constraints.

Analytical frameworks – rationalist approach

Analytic models are based on a rationalistic perspective and assume that the decision makers' cognitive thought-process is logical and is possible to flow and study during the actual decision-making process. *Rational decision making* relates to a time in Utopia where we are able to have all the knowledge about all the possible alternative decisions that are available to us. Problems have to be systematically analysed and decisions are chosen. The model provides clarity and rationality and can be broken down into steps; the chosen decision is then implemented by following a logical step by step approach (Daft, 2009).

There is also the concept of *bounded rationality* (Beach and Connolly, 2005). This recognises the limitations of decision making and that the rationality of individuals is limited by the information available, cognitive limitations and the concept that there is restricted time/resources to make a decision. In this model of decision making, we often seek to find a satisfactory solution rather than the optimal one.

The *garbage can* model concept originates from the theory that solutions and decisions are made and used and then reused. It was developed by Cohen et al. (1972) in relation to how organisational decision making takes place where organisations experience high levels of uncertainty. The garbage can model does not view the decision-making process as a logical sequential process of steps beginning with a problem and ending with a solution. Instead, decisions come as an outcome from almost always totally independent streams of events within such an organisation. It suggests that there are four possible consequences that will result from such a decision-making process: solutions may be proposed for situations where problems do not really exist, choices on decision-making outcomes are made without solving the problem, problems may persist without being solved regardless of the decision made or some problems are solved by the decision making. The garbage can model allows problems to be addressed and choices to be made, but does not necessarily follow a rational process.

The hypothetico-deductive framework

There are several models within this framework but one of the most influential methods of clinical decision making is the hypothetico-deductive that originated in medicine (Elstein et al., 1978) and subsequently applied to nursing (Tanner et al., 1987; Jones, 1988; Taylor, 1997). The other commonly used framework is the cognitive continuum method which was originated by Hammond (1978).

Hypothetico-deductive method

This approach applies both inductive and deductive reasoning methods and clinicians widely rely on this method of decision making (Jensen et al., 2009). Elstein et al. (1978) states that using the hypothetico-deductive model involves four stages:

1. Cue acquisition – Gathering information and clinical data.
2. Hypothesis generation – Listing of 4–6 differential diagnosis.
3. Cue interpretation – Interpretative data (e.g. vital signs, diagnostic testing (e.g. blood sugar measurement) to confirm or refute differential diagnosis).
4. Hypothesis evaluation – weighing up pros and cons of each possible explanation for signs and symptoms and choosing interventions favoured by evidence collected.

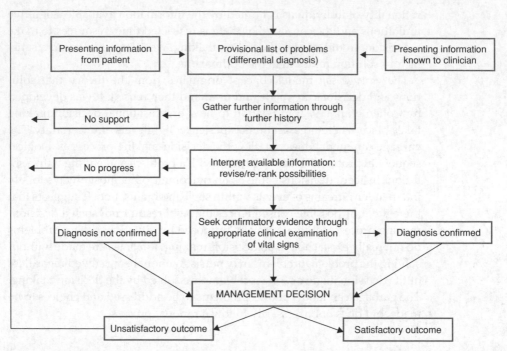

Figure 3.1   Hypothetico-deductive model.

It can be used to rule out the worst case scenario (e.g. myocardial infarction) and allow time for further collection of data from the patient. Time needs to be spent gathering as much information as possible to rule out particular conditions. To rule out the worst case scenario, clinician runs through a list of 'red flag/can't miss' conditions, which may be identified though the intuitive methods. The clinician compares the presenting symptoms which those of his/her 'list' to exclude conditions, initially those that are life-threatening or may lead to a poor outcome for the patient. It can then allow a 'working diagnosis' based on the information found in the patient history taking and assessment, which can be modified based on further information being gained.

If we look at chest pain as an example, using this method a list of competing diagnoses is devised through collating initial cues such as age; weight; various descriptors of pain such as location, duration and intensity. This may lead to preliminary hypotheses of cardiac pain or pain from alternative sources such as respiratory problems, ulcers, indigestion, etc. To rule out cardiac pain, hypotheses will cause the deduction of further data; for example, an ECG, asking questions about previous history and through close observation of the patient's behaviour whilst in pain. The new data provide evidence for or against the competing hypotheses (differential diagnosis) and the cycle continues and the clinical encounter is used to collect information to allow the clinician to determine the most plausible hypothesis, given the evidence. The clinician then investigates further and either gains confirmation on the hypothesis or not. If confirmation is gained, then a decision on treatment/the way forward is devised. If a negative result is gained, then the clinician goes back to gaining more information and then again testing the hypothesis and so on. Figure 3.1 demonstrates this simply through the use of a flow chart.

Using this cognitive strategy means that the clinician considers other possibilities before acting (Croskerry, 2005). It is important, however, that clinicians have a breadth of understanding of pathophysiology in order to be able to include or exclude those related to each particular patient. If only a limited amount of pathophysiology is known, then the clinicians' list will be limited and has a high chance of leading to omissions.

Critical thinking

Using the medical model for history taking (see Chapter 1), consider the following case study and identify which method of decision making is adopted at each question.
A 25 year old male presented with shortness of breath and 'flu-type symptoms'.
   Based on this information what is your immediate impression?
The patient has been unwell for 36 hours with 'flu-type symptoms'. He suffers with asthma and has not taken his ventolin for 24 hours as he has not had time to go to the doctors to get his medication. He has no audible wheeze, equal rise and fall of his chest and hyperventilation. He has no peripheral cyanosis and has a good colour.
   What is your impression now?
   Make a list of differential diagnosis from this information.
   Vital signs reveal;
Pulse rate: 102 beats per minute
Respiratory rate: 29 breaths per minute (hyperventilating)
Blood pressure: 120.90 mmHg
Temperature: 37.9°C
Oxygen saturation: 98% on air
Glasgow Coma Scale: 15/15 (E4, V5 & M6)
   Has this changed your impression?
   Have you narrowed down your differential diagnosis?
   Have you added to your list of differential diagnosis?
   Do you have enough information for the history of presenting complaint?
   What further information is needed?
   Are you certain that your impression may be correct?

On gaining a past medical history, the patient tells you he is asthmatic and insulin dependent diabetic. He takes ventolin as required for his asthma and Insulatard 25 units twice daily. His blood sugar reading is 29 mmol.
Now what is your impression?
How many of you had considered that the patient had a respiratory problem?

The patient in this case study was suffering from diabetic ketosis. This highlights the potential problems that relates to misunderstandings and errors that can occur at different stages of the process. It is important to note that clinical decision making is being able to justify those decisions regardless of the outcome. When linking to history taking (see Chapter 1), you would need to consider more in-depth information regarding his history of presenting complaint as this information is insufficient. You would need to clarify what the 'flu-type' symptoms are, is there any chest pain? Is there any sputum? Or associated symptoms as described by the patient. This is where you can use the mnemonics (see Chapter 1).

Cognitive continuum framework

The *cognitive continuum theory* matches cognitive tasks to the different demands of decisions and the competence of the individual needs to achieve this. This theory is based on the fact that the theories and models already identified within the chapter all have different strengths and weaknesses. Hammond (1978, 1996) joined together the intuition/experimental and analytic/rational decision making and formed the cognitive continuum theory in the belief that different decisions require different approaches. He created a system of different decision-making tasks which range from 'ill structured' to 'well structured' which prompt a response from 'intuition' to 'analysis'. He identified six modes of inquiry, when decisions are made from appropriately matching cognitive tasks to the demands/requirements of the given particular situation. This allows the strengths of each approach to be utilised at the most optimum time.

Figure 3.2 shows how the combined approaches to decision making are blended and changed as the decision tasks change from being well structured to being ill structured. Modes 1 to 3 are more time consuming in obtaining a decision whereas in modes 4 to 6, decision making is much quicker, using tacit knowledge. The choice of mode depends upon the individual being able to perform an assessment in relation to the urgency (e.g. cardiac arrest) and complexity of the situation (e.g. patients with a range of comorbidity conditions making assessment and management difficult).

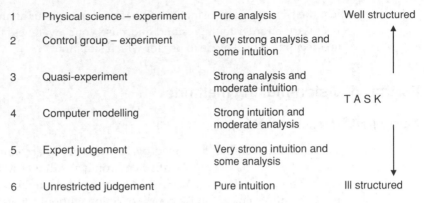

1	Physical science – experiment	Pure analysis	Well structured
2	Control group – experiment	Very strong analysis and some intuition	
3	Quasi-experiment	Strong analysis and moderate intuition	
			TASK
4	Computer modelling	Strong intuition and moderate analysis	
5	Expert judgement	Very strong intuition and some analysis	
6	Unrestricted judgement	Pure intuition	Ill structured

Figure 3.2   Hammond's (1996) Six modes of enquiry.

The cognitive continuum model l was adapted by Hamm (1988) to include system-aided, peer-aided and intuition judgement which are recognised as being used in healthcare (see Figure 3.3). System-aided judgement includes some of the other decision-making models discussed earlier in the chapter and include the use of algorithms, guidelines or protocols to support decision making. Peer-aided judgement involves paramedics discussing probable diagnosis and possible interventions with experienced colleagues and seeking expert advice where it is required. Using more analytical modes does not guarantee that mistakes in decision making will not be made. Errors or mistakes can occur when using research findings

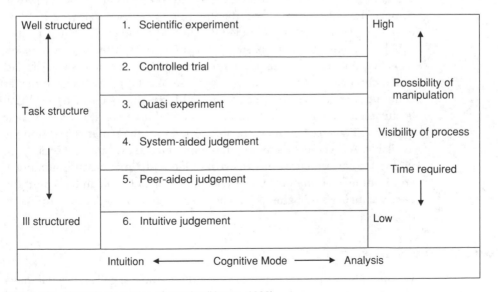

Figure 3.3   Hamm's six modes of enquiry (Hamm, 1988).

just the same as when using intuition. Developing your analytical skills is necessary in order to understand and raise your awareness for when you are deciding which mode to use for which situation.

Further decision-making methods

Naturalistic decision making

This method was first developed by Klein (1999) to account for decision making by experts in time sensitive environments. It was initially used to explain how experienced Fire Ground Commanders could use their expertise to identify and carry out a course of action without generating analyses of options for purposes of comparison. This is based on the premise that often there is not enough time to apply normative choice rules. Instead, experienced decision makers follow recognition of primed decision-making strategy.

This is a model of how people make quick, effective decisions when faced with complex situations. The decision maker picks up on aspects of the situation that leads them to recognise patterns. Depending on the patterns and the decisions that the individual needs to make, the decision maker chooses a single course of action that they think will achieve the outcome required. Klein (1999) suggested that the decision maker would run the script through a mental simulation, based on the mental models the decision maker has developed through experience. This allows the decision maker to idealise how things will follow based on their knowledge through experience. The decision maker compares this against what is known to work. In response to this, if the decision maker thinks that the script will achieve the outcome, they will then pursue the chosen pathway. If, however, they feel that this may not get the desired result or may cause further problems then they alter the script. Following this, if the decision maker feels that this will not meet the requirements then they may even discard it and choose a completely different course of action. The decision maker continues to rehearse the chosen script until they find one which they think is suitable. There is no direct comparison of alternative; it is only as their expertise increases that they are able to identify the patterns and options available. As expertise increases, the chance increases in the first script providing the correct outcome. This works well with time pressure situations, and is quite a natural process; however, it does only take into account the decision maker's thoughts as he/she does not ask for feedback or opinions of others.

Group decision making

We often think that making decisions with a group of colleagues will have great benefits, yet evidence shows that there are benefits and detriments with group decision making (Tindale, 2004). If a group reaches a consensus decision, then it can be easier to implement the decision within an organisation as opposed to an individual enforcing their solution (Amason, 1996). Positively, competition between group members can lead to better decisions/solutions being imagined (Huber, 1984) and groups making decisions can avoid dictatorships (Bainbridge, 2002). Yet, there are some disadvantages; individuals can be prone to go along with the dominant theory of the majority which is called the phenomenon of groupthink (Janis, 1972). People think in different ways and hold different beliefs. There is a potential for conflict and for individuals to manipulate others into their way of thinking, so that they get the desired response. Members may not always put the same level of thinking into the decision (Hirokawa et al., 1996) and group decisions can result in no decision or riskier decisions – as no one person is held to account for the decision being made.

> ## Discussion point
>
> Can you think of clinical incidents when you can apply this method of decision making?

Tools to support clinical decision making

Clinical guidelines

Clinical guidelines are readily available to help guide clinical practice and the National Institute for Clinical Excellence is continually increasing it guidance. One drawback of guidelines is their timeliness. Guidelines do take some considerable time to develop as they draw on a wide breadth of up to date evidence. However, as evidence is being produced regularly, then guidance/guideline can only be as up to date as the available evidence was when it was produced. This means that as soon as new evidence becomes available, then the guidance/guideline may not now be considered to be the best practice as the new evidence may conflict or supersede what was previously written. New guidance/guidelines based on this new evidence will then take some time for it to be rewritten or reproduced. One example of this is the Joint Royal College Association Liaison Committee (JRCALC) guidelines. The current version was produced in 2006 and yet much more evidence has since been published – for example, the British Thoracic Society (2010) and Resuscitation Council UK (2010).

Protocols

Protocols are rigid directions that follow the best practice laid down in guidelines to help clinicians apply the appropriate intervention within their organisation. Traditionally, it has been thought that paramedics make most of their clinical decisions by following the appropriate protocol from memory. However, it has now been suggested that paramedics are likely to use other thinking strategies to make clinical decisions as this is probably not a sufficient explanation for how paramedics make decisions (Bigham et al., 2011). (See Chapter 5 for further reading on guidelines and protocols in practice.)

Algorithms

These are extremely useful in decision making; they are developed from research evidence and patient data. Usually clinicians commit algorithms to memory (or have cue cards) and use them when presented with a suitable situation. A classic example of this is using the Advanced Cardiac Life Support algorithms to determine treatment for a patient in cardiac arrest (Resuscitation Council UK, 2010).

Decision trees

Decision trees are similar to algorithms in nature and provide a decision support tool that uses a tree like graph or model of decision and possible outcomes/consequences. They are commonly used to identify a way forward to reach a likely goal, clearly laying out the problems so that all options can be explored. They allow you to focus on the possible consequences of a decision and provide the framework to identify the outcomes and probability of achieving them based on the existing information.

Decision matrix

This tool is a quantitative technique to rank multidimensional options of an option set; for example, the risk matrixes used in risk assessments. This involves establishing set criteria which can be used so that potential options can be scored and summed in order to gain a total score which can then be ranked. It can help in the subjective opinions about one thing versus another can be made more objective. However, ultimately how you score the different options can remain subjective.

The Bayesian approach

This approach to decision making uses elements of Bayesian probability theory using intelligence, mathematical assumptions and graphical analysis together as a decision-making tool. All possible causes and effect linkages are described and reduced using algorithms. This results in a reduction of complexity of the problem requiring a decision and results in an outcome. However, this is not often used in healthcare, being used more so with computer systems.

Clinical decision-making skills

So far, we have discussed decision-making theories, models and tools to support clinical decision making. Whilst these help you to structure and justify your decision making, this may not be sufficient. The collection of information, beliefs and observation is also essential to build a picture of the patient upon which to base a decision. Thus, it can be suggested that in order to do this, knowledge, experiences and the ability to think critically are the most important factors that will influence decision making. The knowledge a paramedic brings to the diagnostic task plays a critical role in determining how the problem will be interpreted and which items of clinical information will be attended to.

Critical thinking

Consider the following case scenario (based on a real incident) and think about your answers to the questions before moving onto the next stage. A 10 year old male presents with abdominal pain and vomiting for the past two days. He is pale and lethargic. No previous medical history, as he is normally fit and well. No current medications.
His vital signs are:

Respiratory rate: 29 breaths per minute and rapid
Oxygen saturation levels: 98% on air
Pulse rate: 130 beats per minute
Blood pressure: 110/80 mmHg
Temperature: 38.0°C
Capillary refill time: 3 seconds
Glasgow Coma Scale: 15/15 (Eye 4, Verbal 5, Motor 6)

What are your thoughts as to the potential diagnosis of this patient? What is the probability of this history relating to a gastrointestinal problem? What is the probability of the vital signs indicating hypovolaemia secondary to excessive fluid loss? Would you consider other differential diagnosis?

Further assessment revealed this young boy had a blood sugar reading of 29 mmol.

With this additional information, what are your thoughts to the potential diagnosis of this patient? Are your differential diagnoses the same or do you have other potential diagnosis? How many of you considered diabetic ketoacidosis?

The working diagnosis for this child was diabetic ketoacidosis secondary to undiagnosed type I diabetes. On further questioning, from his mother it was revealed that she had noticed that he had excessive thirst and that he had lost weight. His mother thought this was due to increased exercise activity. Excessive thirst and weight loss are common symptoms for uncontrolled type 1 diabetes. From your observation of the patient, his high respiratory rate was a Kussmaul's respiration, which is a common symptom of diabetic ketoacidosis. Would you have connected the signs and symptoms and history to this diagnosis?

In contrast to the previous case study, the working diagnosis is the same; however, the clinical presentations are very different. When we make decisions as previously stated, it does rely on a collated variety of evidence and in both cases, the history of presenting complaint, past medical history and diagnostic test (blood sugar reading) was vital to achieve the appropriate outcome. This would have also included the use of standards, guidelines and/or protocols that would also be used to ensure that you practiced safely, professionally and lawfully to achieve the appropriate outcomes, thus supporting your clinical decision making. When making choices in decision making, the knowledge we draw upon comes from a variety of sources such as shared knowledge, life experiences, expertise of others and research evidence through the use of guidelines etc. Sackett et al. (2000) support this and states

'the integration of best research evidence with clinical expertise and patient values are used to facilitate clinical decision making . . . '. (p. 1)

Patients may come with straightforward problems or they may be multiple and very complex and it is important to identify and prioritise the most important by having the ability to sift or analyse the evidence and respond flexibly to them. The process of critical thinking is oriented towards making judgements about many situations encountered on a daily basis. At the same time, you need to be able to see the broader picture and engage the skills of analysis, evaluation and interpretation and the integration of knowledge and skills are insufficient alone. The ability to think critically builds the foundation for clinical decision making and will assist you to think beyond routines and protocols. To be an effective critical thinkers, you must also have the necessary attributes, habits of mind and attitudes to use knowledge and complement the skills (Profetto-McGrath, 2003). These dispositions would include the following:

- Decision making/problem solving skills
- Inquisitiveness
- Well informed
- Open minded
- Questioning skills
- Confidence

Questioning is a skill that can be learned and a service to activate critical thinking and to be an indicator of its use. Questions can be used to challenge what is heard, observed, read, and experienced in practice. Well-articulated questions are important as they direct you to the necessary evidence, reveal gaps in the present evidence, assist in gathering the evidence necessary to solve patients' problem or to support best practice (Foster, 2004; Kee and Bickle, 2004; Twibell et al., 2005). Chapter 1 (History Taking) offers further information on questioning skills and to be read in conjunction with Chapter 2 (Consultation and Communication Skills).

Open-mindedness is the ability to form an opinion or revise it in the light of evidence and argument. Sellman (2003) considers open-mindedness as a virtue for professional practice. In opposition, closed-mindedness will hold firm to a position or idea regardless of what the evidence indicates and discusses the notion that he or she may be incorrect. For example, someone who is open minded will be open to the currency of a guideline as well as its suitability in the provision of care to a patient and is likely to consider a number of options. Alternatively, someone who is closed minded will be quick to follow the guideline despite its questionable validity and individual patient care needs.

It is evident that critical thinkers are able to explore all forms of evidence and make reasoned judgements as to their suitability to be applied to the current situation. They must also be aware of personal biases (this is discussed later in the chapter) that may influence the decision reach. It is evident that critical thinking and clinical decision making require a range of knowledge and skills. The American Philosophical Association (1990) captures the essence of a critical thinker as they state a critical thinker as a

> habitually inquisitive, well informed, trustful of reason, open minded, flexible, fair minded in evaluation, honest in facing personal biases, prudent in making judgments, willing to reconsider, clear about issues, orderly in complex matters, diligent in seeking relevant information, reasonable in the selection of criteria, focussed on enquiry and persistent in seeking results which are as process, as the subject and the circumstances of inquiry permit. (p. 3)

Uncertainty within critical decision making

In clinical decision making, when predicting outcomes for patients, we have to remember that prediction can be inconsistent. Patients can be selective in what they tell us, old knowledge has to be replaced and research can be flawed; therefore, critical decision making always involves discriminating between the following:

- Certainty
- Near certainty
- Degree in uncertainty

Critical thinking

Consider the following questions

1. If a decision is to be considered rational, then surely some knowledge of what the future might look like after the decision is made is required?
2. How many of us can truthfully say what the future is going to look like?
3. How many of us thought something predictable is going to happen, only to have something unexpected take its place?

Decision making is inherently uncertain (Tversky and Kahnemann, 1974). Within the pre-hospital setting, it is common to have incomplete knowledge about the patient, the history or the current situation. This incomplete knowledge is referred to as uncertainty (Sanderson and Gruen, 2006) and uncertainty is considered to be inherent within decision making in healthcare (Thompson and Dowding, 2009). What is vitally important is that as a clinician you identify the uncertainty, and where possible you act on it. This is even more difficult when, according to Sanderson and Gruen (2006), uncertainty implies that you know what possible outcomes might be, but have no information about the likelihood of each and risk implies knowledge about the probability of each outcome. Furthermore, the causes of uncertainty can be due to one of the following:

- Ignorance; for example, an area of the patient's history is not understood in sufficient detail or contraindications of a particular drug treatment are not fully understood or the latest treatment is not understood by the clinician.
- Incomplete information; for example, the patient did not inform you about part of their medical history, which impacts on their current care/presenting complaint.
- The inability to predict the moves of other parties involved; for example, if you were in a rapid response vehicle and you were waiting on an ambulance crew for assistance and did not know how long they were going to take to arrive at your location.
- Measurement errors; for example, you checked a patient's blood glucose reading but did not realise they had a substance on their finger which gave a false reading.

When confronted with a situation where there is a degree of uncertainty or at least a situation when you are aware there may be a degree of uncertainty, it is suggested that asking the correct questions is key (Adair, 2010). This may, however, not necessarily mean asking the patient, but it may need a time of inner reflection to ask oneself the questions, but this does require one to have made some sort of decision in order to know which questions to ask. This is of course compounded when faced with a time critical situation.

How do you measure the uncertainty?

It is common to define and describe risks using probabilities and probability distributions (Aven, 2010); however, these probabilities can camouflage uncertainties (Rosa, 1998; Aven, 2010). Probability is a measure or representation of the uncertainty associated with our decision making. Thompson and Bland (2009) cited two different definitions of probability:

- The ideas that probability is an expression of a subjective degree of belief
- The notion that probability represents frequency of a phenomenon in a sample of observations

It is described by Thompson and Bland (2009) as being represented numerically; odds, however, can range from 0 to infinity – representing the ratio of the chance of something happening to the change of something not happening. For example, if we have a phenomenon of 0.75 (75%) chance of something happening and 0.25 (25%) chance of it not happening (0.75/0.25 or written 3 to 1 or 3:1), odds mean that you will have three occurrences of it happening for every one chance it does not occur (Thompson and Bland, 2009). However, in reality, we often use language such as 'rare' or 'unlikely' or 'good chance' when describing uncertainty, rather than the probability of 0 to 100% or 0 to 1 – with 0 being no chance at all of it happening and 1 when it is certain that the phenomenon you are interested in will occur (Thompson and Dowding, 2009). These qualitative expressions of certainty or uncertainty may be more comfortable especially when individuals have no real idea of the size/measure of the relevant risk. Perhaps it is easier to use when a chance can be defined exactly, when there is a level of statistical ability and the outcome is predictable within limits. Unfortunately, within healthcare, this is not always the case.

Arnoldi (2009), however, talks about a distinction between objective and subjective probability (citing legal theory abandoning numerical probability theory and turning instead to conceptual understanding of subjective probability – most notably, the idea of proof beyond reasonable doubt). In some cases, estimation can rely entirely on a calculation. In other cases, however, we may be estimating a quantity which is observable, based on introspective observations or could involve undertaking measurements with values that can be applied to the external world. Confidence reports ('I believe the chances of rain tomorrow in Stafford is 80%') are an example of such measurements, as are estimates based on perception such as the loudness of crying or how many tablets are scattered on the floor. In each situation, however, in order to be confident in them, we need to ask how well calibrated these individual measurements are and was any of the measurements flawed in any way.

Recognising the presence of uncertainty can be viewed as constructive (Standing, 2010) and sits firmly with being an accountable practitioner (HCPC, 2012). It is in fact an aspect of lifelong learning and the continuation of self education (HCPC, 2012).

Ultimately, all decisions will be made under some level of uncertainty. It is a continuum with polar ends of certainty and uncertainty. Decisions will fall somewhere within this. Intelligent decision making is based on some knowledge of size and nature of risk (Koontz and Weihrich, 2008) and sits firmly with acknowledging this risk.

Factors affecting your decision making

You may consider that all of your decisions are completely unbiased; however, think again. Our life experiences will completely impact on how we view and make decisions; these are often referred to as 'lenses' through which we view things.

> **Discussion point**
>
> Consider the analgesia you would administer for the two presenting problems given in the examples:
>
> A 40 year old male with severe abdominal pain.
> A 40 year old male with severe abdominal pain – known intravenous drug user (IVDU)
> How would those three words (IVDU) affect your decision making?

Human tendency leads us to often base a judgement or decision on a flawed or poor perception of our understanding of data or events. These can be referred to as biases or lenses through which we view the world. Some of the commonly encountered biases/lenses are described below:

Confirmation bias: misinterpretation of data so that it suites the person making the decision (Nickerson, 1998).
Optimism bias: when you are over optimistic about what will happen as a result of the planned action.
Anchoring: relying heavily on a single piece of information when making a decision which can increase the risks associated with the decision.

Availability bias: basing decisions on sources of information that can be easily recalled, rejecting what could be potentially more important information without considering it in depth.

Representativeness: making judgements based on a seemingly representative known sample (for example, to make a decision based on a similar task) also where probability of events are estimated based on those of comparable event that is known to the decision maker.

Selective perception: to give undue or higher importance to data that support your own views. To hear what we want to hear will result in a skewed perception of risk.

Loss aversion: to give preference to avoiding loss over making gain – for example, over caution might result in an increase in the probability of risk.

Information bias: to seek as much data as possible prior to making a decision, which results in being swamped by data that does not improve the quality of the decision.

Omission bias: where there is a tendency to judge decisions that cause direct harm to be worse than those that cause indirect harm (Baron, 2000).

Status quo bias: results in a preference for omission or inaction and can lead to the decision maker choosing the risks and benefits of the status quo even when the relative risks and benefits of a change (making a decision) are superior. These stem from heuristics 'rule of thumb' (Bostrom and Ord, 2006).

Conservatism and inertia: the unwillingness to change our thought patterns from one we have used previously even when faced with a new situation or fitting situations in order to make them fit.

Experiential limitations: the unwillingness or inability to look beyond what we have experienced in the past, instead we choose to reject the unfamiliar option.

Selective perception: is when we actively screen out information we do not believe to be salient or relevant to the situation (Parcon, 2007).

Choice supportive: distorting memories of previously chosen and rejected options to make the chosen options seem relatively more acceptable (Parcon, 2007).

Wishful thinking or optimism: seeing things in a positive light, which can distort our thinking and perception of the situation (Parcon, 2007).

Role fulfilment: conforming to decision making expectations that others (our peers, colleagues, line managers) have of someone in our position (Parcon, 2007).

Groupthink: can be referred to as peer pressure, where we conform to the opinions held by the group rather than stand alone with your own opinion.

Faulty generalisations: in order to simplify a complex situation, we group things and people and make simplifying generalisations (Parcon, 2007).

Premature termination bias: accepting the first solution that may appear to work.

Inertia: unwillingness to change thought patterns.

Source credibility bias: being inclined to accept a statement, suggestion or decision by someone we like; for example, a colleague who we consider to be more senior or indeed guidelines from professional organisations.

Belief/behavioural bias: propensity to make decisions while being influenced by underlying belief e.g. optimism, over confidence, illusion of control (Chira et al., 2008).

Distinction bias: in a group or joint evaluation of a decision, people incorporate values of the group but may experience outcome individually and can give higher weight/importance to a given criteria in the group rather than as an individual experiencing it (Hsee and Zhang, 2004).

Projection bias: where decision makers exaggerate the degree to which future requirements will resemble the current needs.

Hindsight bias: person uses hindsight knowledge of previous events to assign a higher weight to those same outcomes in future events.

Outcome bias: people believe good decision equate to good outcomes and vice versa but evidence shows this is not so, can lead to revamping good decision process in response to bad outcome (Reason, 2007).

As can be seen, there is a plethora of information which the decision maker needs to be aware of when making a decision, which is magnified when time is at a premium and a quick decision has to be made. These include being conscious of your decisions wherever possible and consider alternatives. In this way, you counter the perceived 'facts' and avoid being led down a line that you 'expect' from your first perceptions. He also suggests that because memory is highly contextual, the background of any situation may have an impact on how we see it. Be critical of research, correlation does not necessarily equal causation. Just because there is a correlation between obesity and chest pain of myocardial origin does not mean that this is the case, it is just more likely. Think about your bias, how it may affect your decision making, try to think broadly about if and when bias may come into play in your decision making. Otherwise, alternatively through which lens you are viewing the situation when faced with a decision-making scenario. Marcus (2008) also suggests that humans are better at concrete goals, so try to see your decision making in these terms. Marcus (2008) also indicates that weighing the costs of the decision against its benefits has important implications, but is difficult to do, at the time, so it is beneficial to be reflective. Looking back on your decision making maintains its conscious quality and in the same vein, imagining that someone is going to spot check our work means that humans make more cognitive effort. Try to distance yourself, be aware of the competing influences on your decision making, and beware of the vivid, personal and anecdotal stories especially of peers or people we might feel are better qualified. Be careful of your information sources, are you being manipulated? Remember that not all decisions are equal, and therefore do not warrant in-depth deliberation. Make a decision! This will get easier with time. Finally, try to be rational, try to work out from first principles – if you understand the context of the decision, then the rational decision should be the right one, and if challenged can be robustly defended.

Summary

It can be seen from the above that there are many theories, framework and tools to support practitioners in the decision-making process. We have attempted to illustrate some of the commonly used frameworks through the use of clinical exemplars. Within the pre-hospital, emergency and urgent care environment, patients along the age continuum present with a wide range of clinical conditions from simple to complex clinical presentations. It is apparent that not one model will fit all and different methods will need to be utilised in different situations. Clinical decision making is a complex process but it is one which the individual practitioner must have the necessary skills and insight into due to the concept of accountability in practice. The more knowledgeable and aware the practitioner is of their decision-making process, the more able they are to understand how and why particular decisions have been made. This will assist the practitioner in their decision-making processes when decisions are being made in relation to patient care delivery, when writing reports or adverse incident forms and also when sharing your skills and knowledge to new practitioners or students.

References

Adair, J. (2010) *Decision Making and Problem Solving Strategies: 66 (Creating Success)*. Kogan Page, London.

Amason, A.C. (1996) Distinguishing the effects of functional and dysfunctional conflicts on strategic decision making: researching a paradox for top management teams. *Academy Management Journal*, **39**(1), 123–148.

American Philosophical Association (1990) *Critical Thinking: A Statement of Expert Consensus for Purposes of Educational Assessment and Instruction*. The California Academic Press, Salt Lake City, VT.

Arnoldi, J. (2009) *Risk*. Polity Press, Cambridge.

Aven, T. (2010) *Misconceptions of Risk*. John Wiley & Sons Ltd, Chichester.

Bainbridge, S.M. (2002) Why a board? Group decision making in corporate governance. *Vanderbilt Law Review*, **55**(1), 1–55.

Baron, J. (2000) *Thinking and Deciding*. Cambridge University Press, Cambridge.

Beach, L.R. & Connolly, T. (2005) *The Psychology of Decision Making: People in Organizations*. Sage Publications Series, London.

Benner, P. (1984) *From Novice to Expert. Excellence and Power in Clinical Nursing Practice*. Addison-Wesley Publishing, Boston, MA.

Benner, P. & Tanner, C. (1987) Clinical judgment: how nurses use intuition. *American Journal of Nursing*, **87**(1), 23–31.

Benner, P., Tanner, C.A. & Chesla, C.A. (1996) *Expertise in Nursing Practice: Caring, Clinical Judgment and Ethics*. Springer, New York.

Bigham, B.L., Bull, E., Morrison, M., et al. (2011) Patient safety in emergency medical services: executive summary and recommendations from the Niagara Summit. *Canadian Association of Emergency Physicians (CJEM)*, **13**(1), 13–18.

Bostrom, N. & Ord, T. (2006) The reversal test: eliminating status quo bias in applied ethics. *Ethics*, **116**(4), 656–679.

British Thoracic Society (2010) *British Thoracic Society Guidelines*. Available from www.brit-thoracic.org.uk/guidelines.aspx (accessed June 2012).

Buckingham, C.D. & Adams, A. (2000) Classifying clinical decision making: a unifying approach. *Journal of Advanced Nursing*, **32**(4), 981–989.

Carnevelli, D.L., Mitchell, P.H., Woods, N.F. & Tanner, C.A. (1984) *Diagnostic Reasoning in Nursing*. Lippincott, Philadelphia.

Carper, B. (1978) Fundamental patterns of knowing in nursing. *Advances in Nursing Science*, **1**(1), 13–23.

Chira, I., Adams, M. & Thornton, B. (2008) Behavioural bias within the decision making process. *Journal of Business and Economics Research*, **6**(8), 11–18.

Cioffi, J. (1997) Heuristics, servants to intuition, in clinical decision-making. *Journal of Advanced Nursing*, **26**(1), 203–208.

Cohen, M., March, J. & Olsen, J. (1972) A garbage can model of organisational choice. *Administrative Science Quarterly*, **17**(1), 1–25.

Croskerry, P. (2005) The theory and practice of clinical decision-making. *Canadian Journal of Anesthesia*, **6**(52), R1–R8.

Daft, R. (2009) *Organization Theory and Design*. South-Western Cengage Learning, Stanford, CT.

Elstein, A.S., Shulman, L.S. & Sprafka, S.A. (1978) *Medical Problem Solving: An Analysis of Clinical Reasoning*. Harvard University Press, London.

Field, P.A. (1987) The impact of nursing theory on the clinical decision making process. *Journal of Advanced Nursing*, **12**(5), 563–571.

Ford, J.A.G., Trygstad-Durland, L.N. & Nelms, B.C. (1979) *Applied Decision Making for Nurses*. Mosby, St. Louis.

Foster, R.L. (2004) Challenges in teaching evidence-based practice. *Journal for Specialists in Pediatric Nursing*, **9**(3), 75–76.

Gigerenzer, G., Todd, P.M. & ABC Research Group (1999) *Simple Heuristics That Make us Smart*. Oxford University Press, New York.

Goleman, D. (2002) *Business: The Ultimate Resource*. Bloomsbury Publications, London.

Grobe, S.J., Drew, J.A. & Fonteyn, M.E. (1988) A descriptive analysis of experience nurses' clinical reasoning during a planned task. *Research in Nursing and Health*, **14**(4), 305–314.

Hamm, R.M. (1988) Clinical intuition and clinical analysis: expertise and the cognitive continuum. In: *Professional Judgment: A Reader in Clinical Decision Making* (eds J. Dowie & A. Elstein). Cambridge University Press, Cambridge.

Hammond, K.R. (1964) An approach to the study of clinical inferences in nursing: Part II. *Nursing Research*, **13**(4), 315–319.

Hammond, K.R. (1978) *Judgment and Decision in Public Policy Formation*. Westview Press, Boulder.

Hammond, K.R. (1996) *Human Judgment and Social Policy: Irreducible Uncertainty, Inevitable Error, Unavoidable Injustice*. Oxford University Press, New York.

Health and Care Professions Council (2012) *Standards of Conduct, Performance and Ethics*. Health and Care Professions Council, London.

Hirokawa, R., Erbert, L. & Hurst, A. (1996) Communication and group decision making effectiveness. In: *Communication and Group Decision Making*, 2nd edn (eds R.Y. Hirokawa & M.S. Poole), pp. 260–300. Sage Publications, London.

Hsee, C.K. & Zhang, J. (2004) Distinction bias: misrepresentation and mischoice due to joint evaluation. *Journal of Personality & Social Psychology*, **86**(5), 680–695.

Huber, G. (1984) Issues in the design of group decision support systems. *Management Information Systems Quarterly*, **8**(3), 195–204.

Janis, I. (1972) *Victims of Group Think*. Houghton Mifflin, Boston.

Jensen, J.L., Croskerry, P. & Travers, A.H. (2009) Paramedic clinical decision making during high acuity emergency calls: design and methodology of a Delphi study. *BMC Emergency Medicine*, **9**(17), 1–4.

Jones, J.A. (1988) Clinical reasoning in nursing. *Journal of Advanced Nursing*, **13**(2), 185–192.

Kahneman, D. & Tversky, A. (2000) *Choice, Values and Frames*. Cambridge University Press, Cambridge.

Kee, F. & Bickle, I. (2004) Critical thinking and critical appraisal: the chicken and the egg? *Quarterly Journal of Medicine*, **97**(9), 609–614.

Klein, G. (1999) *Sources of Power: How People Make Decisions*. MIT Press, London.

Koontz, H. & Weihrich, H. (2008) *Essentials of Management: An International Perspective*. McGraw Hill, New Delhi.

Luker, K. & Kendrick, M. (1992) An exploratory study of the sources of influence on clinical decisions of community nurses. *Journal of Advanced Nursing*, **17**(4), 457–466.

Marcus, G. (2008) *Kluge: The Haphazard Construction of the Human Mind*. Houghton Mifflin, Boston.

Nickerson, S. (1998) Confirmation bias: a ubiquitous phenomenon in many guises. *Review of General Psychology*, **2**(2), 175–220.

Parcon, P. (2007) *Develop Your Decision Making Skills*. Lotus Books, Canada.

Profetto-McGrath, J. (2003) The relationship of critical thinking skills and critical thinking dispositions of baccalaureate nursing students. *Journal of Advanced Nursing*, **43**(6), 569–577.

Radwin, L.E. (1990) Research on diagnostic reasoning in nursing. *Nursing Diagnosis*, **1**(2), 70–77.

Reason, J. Professor Emeritus, University of Manchester (2007) Presentation entitled *Managing The Risks of Organizational Accidents*.

Resuscitation Council UK (2010) *Resuscitation Guidelines*. Resuscitation Council UK, London.

Rosa, E.A. (1998) Metatheoretical foundations for post-normal risk. *Journal of Risk Research*, **1**(1), 15–44.

Sackett, D.L., Straus, S.E., Richardson, W.C., Rosenberg, W. & Haynes, R.M. (2000) *Evidence-Based Medicine: How to Practice and Teach EBM*. Churchill Livingstone, New York.

Sanderson, C. & Gruen, R. (2006) *Analytical Models for Decision Making*. Open University Press, Maidenhead.

Sellman, D. (2003) Open-mindedness: a virtue for professional practice. *Nursing Philosophy*, **4**(1), 17–24.

Standing, M. (ed.) (2010) *Clinical Judgement and Decision-Making: In Nursing and Interprofessional Healthcare*. Open University Press, Maidenhead.

Tanner, C.A., Padrick, K.P., Westfall, U.E. & Putzier, D.J. (1987) Diagnostic reasoning strategies of nurses and nursing students. *Nursing Research*, **36**(6), 358–363.

Taylor, C. (1997) Problem solving in clinical nursing practice. *Journal of Advanced Nursing*, **26**(2), 329–336.

Thompson, C. & Bland, M. (2009) Probability: the language of uncertainty. In: *Essential Decision Making and Clinical Judgment for Nurses* (eds C. Thompson & D. Dowding). Churchill Livingstone, Edinburgh.

Thompson, C. & Dowding, D. (2009) *Clinical Decision Making and Judgement in Nursing*. Churchill Livingstone, Edinburgh.

Tindale, R.S. (2004) Group performance and decision making. *Annual Review of Psychology*, **55**, 623–655.

Tversky, A. & Kahnemann, D. (1974) Judgment under uncertainty: heuristics and biases. *Science*, **185**(4157), 1124–1131.

Twibell, R., Ryan, M. & Hermiz, M. (2005) Faculty perceptions of critical thinking in student clinical experiences. *Journal of Nursing Education*, **44**(2), 71–79.

4 Evidence Based Practice

Louise Perkinton[1] and Val Nixon[2]

[1] Faculty of Education, Health and Sciences, University of Derby, Derby, UK
[2] Faculty of Health Sciences, Staffordshire University, Stafford, UK

Introduction

There are many reasons why healthcare practitioners in paramedic, emergency and urgent care should consider the concept of evidence based practice (EBP). The amount of knowledge available to practitioners and to patients in recent years has vastly increased, alongside the emphasis on quality of care and litigation in healthcare. These all point directly to the need for practitioners to use the best available evidence to inform their practice. After considering the background to EBP, this chapter brings together the skills required to identify, evaluate and use evidence effectively in everyday practice. There has been much debate about what constitutes evidence for healthcare practice in recent years (Hewitt-Taylor, 2003; Rycroft-Malone et al., 2004a) and the various potential evidence sources available to practitioners are explored to enable access to appropriate evidence, relevant to paramedic, emergency and urgent care practice.

Critical appraisal of evidence is a key skill that practitioners need to develop in order to have confidence in taking forward recommendations for change based on evidence (Barker, 2010). There are a number of different approaches that can be adopted and these are discussed through the application of useful appraisal tools. The process of EBP also informs the development of clinical guidelines and protocols and the development and employment of these in practice are explored, with consideration of both the advantages and disadvantages of their use for practitioners. The chapter concludes with the practical application of employing evidence in practice, potential barriers to EBP, and how it resonates with professional standards and frameworks.

Professional Practice in Paramedic, Emergency and Urgent Care, First Edition. Edited by Val Nixon.
© 2013 John Wiley & Sons, Ltd. Published 2013 by John Wiley & Sons, Ltd.

Historical background of evidence based practice

The concept of EBP originated with the work of Archie Cochrane in the 1970s (Cochrane, 1972, 1979). His emphasis was on the medical profession and their failure to organise evidence in a readily accessible way and to use this to guide their practice to ensure that it is appropriate and effective. Cochrane argued that healthcare resources should be used effectively to provide care that has been proven to give the best outcome. He also encouraged the use of evidence and recognised randomised controlled trials (RCTs) as the most reliable source of evidence. RCTs are seen as one of the simplest yet most powerful research methods used in clinical research. In 1979, he criticised his own profession of medicine for not having organised critical summaries of RCTs by specialty to inform practice.

The development of systematic reviews of RCTs in perianal medicine during the 1970s and 1980s led to the opening of the Cochrane Centre in Oxford in 1992, followed by the establishment of the Cochrane Collaboration in 1993. The Cochrane Centre is now an international organisation that focusses on producing systematic reviews of primary research in human healthcare and health policy. As a result, the Cochrane Centre plays a leading role in developing and promoting evidence based healthcare. An interesting timeline (that can be accessed at http://www.cochrane.org/about-us/history) details the numerous achievements of this collaboration in promoting the evidence base for care. Notable milestones include the launch of the Cochrane library and internet access to the database of systematic reviews in 1996. In 1998, systematic reviews were recognised as academically important research by the UK medical colleges. The Cochrane Library is freely available in many countries, and access arrangements are detailed at the following location: http://www.thecochranelibrary.com/view/0/FreeAccess.html.

Cochrane reviews are organised by discipline into review groups or fields of practice. Two notable groups of relevance for health professionals in paramedic, emergency and urgent care are the Cochrane Injury Group (CIG) – established in 1997 (available at http://injuries.cochrane.org/) – and the Nursing Care Field group – established in 2009 (available at http://cncf.cochrane.org/home). The CIG groups have reviewed a wide range of evidence on the effects of interventions, treatment and rehabilitation in relation, for example, abdominal trauma, chest trauma, head injuries and poisoning. Robertson-Malt (2010) also presents a summary of a Cochrane systematic review of advanced trauma life support for hospital staff. Alongside Cochrane reviews, the development of evidence based medicine (EBM) has also been rapid over the past 10 years and has been led by Professor David Sackett. In the 1990s, other healthcare professions, notably nursing began to embrace the principles of evidence based care and the term evidence based practice (EBP) emerged (Barker, 2010).

The Joanna Briggs Institute (JBI, 2011), established in 1996, was another important collaborative organisation and source of evidence for healthcare and had its origins in nursing. Presently, the membership has evolved and includes medical and allied health researchers, clinicians, academics and quality managers. The JBI collaborates internationally with over 70 organisations to provide reliable evidence to inform clinical decision making at the point of care. More information about the background to EBP can be found at the Cochrane and JBI websites (see Box 4.1). The JBI offer guidance on three main aspects of EBP which are

1. Accessing reliable evidence
2. Evaluating that evidence
3. Implementing it in practice

Box 4.1   Background to EBP

For more information about the origins of EBP, see the websites of the Cochrane Collaboration and the JBI at
  http://www.cochrane.org/
  http://www.joannabriggs.edu.au/Home

These stages will be discussed later in the chapter. Some of their resources are freely available to individuals, for example, best practice information sheets, but a number of resources are restricted to JBI members.

What is evidence based practice?

The most widely cited definition in the literature when considering EBP is essentially a definition of EBM which is

'The conscientious, explicit and judicious use of current best evidence in making decisions about the care of individual patients. The practice of evidence based medicine means integrating individual clinical expertise with the best available external clinical evidence from systematic research'. (Sackett et al., 1996, p. 71)

This definition emphasises the need to combine the individual clinician's expertise with external evidence from systematic research in decision making, the clinician judging the evidence that is appropriate to use in their field of practice. This definition is adopted and/or adapted by many authors (Ingersoll, 2000; Hewitt-Taylor, 2003; Shapiro, 2007; Fitzpatrick, 2007a) to define EBP, but there are potential problems with the use of this definition in healthcare professions allied to medicine. Firstly, systematic research may not always be available to support practice and secondly, in addition to clinician expertise and research, we need to recognise the importance of patient involvement in their care.

Ingersoll (2000, p. 152) has suggested an alternative definition for evidence based nursing, which acknowledges these issues and defines evidence based nursing practice as

> the conscientious, explicit and judicious use of theory-derived, research-based information in making decisions about care delivery to individuals or groups of patients and in consideration of individual needs and preferences.

This can be equally applied to allied health professions and this point is also taken up by Donohoe and Blaber (2008) who debate the challenge of making the patient and patient choice central in emergency care. Muir Gray (1997, p. 3) suggests that evidence based healthcare is simply, 'doing the right things right' or

> an approach to decision making in which the clinician uses the best evidence available, in consultation with the patient, to decide upon the option which suits the patient best. (Muir Gray, 1997, p. 9)

Why do we need to use evidence based practice?

Few practitioners would argue with the concept of their care being based on evidence; however, employing an EBP approach requires striving always to use the best evidence that is available and accessible at any given time. Whilst adopting such an approach, it is an appropriate response to the many drivers behind the EBP movement. A major driver for the growth of EBP has been the clinical governance agenda in the National Health Service (NHS).

First introduced in 1998, the process of clinical governance placed a central focus on quality in the NHS, by providing a framework within which the practitioners can operate to improve and safeguard standards of care. It acts as an umbrella term for activities aimed at quality improvement, to include research, clinical audit, service reviews and development of clinical guidelines (RCN, 2003). Within this umbrella activity, clinical effectiveness is seen as the process of development of guidelines for best practice; transferring these into practice settings and evaluating their impact through, for example, clinical audit. Box 4.2 illustrates some drivers for the use of EBP in healthcare which range from those that can be identified for individual practitioners to those that apply across organisations and professions.

Box 4.2   **Drivers for the use of evidence based practice**

Vast increase in the amount of information available to practitioners
Recognised gap between best evidence and practice
Greater emphasis on effective and efficient use of resources
Increasing emphasis on accountability amongst healthcare profession-
  als, partly due to a rise in litigation in healthcare
Increased emphasis on improving the quality of care delivery
Patients and clients well informed through improved access to evidence
Need for interprofessional learning and transferable lessons between
  disciplines

Many healthcare reforms that have been introduced since 1990 were aimed towards improving the standard of care delivery and to develop and implement strategies to improve equity of access to healthcare services which are underpinned by EBP. The National Service Frameworks (NSFs) and National Institution of Health Clinical Excellence (NIHCE) both set clear quality requirements for care. This is based on the best available evidence of what treatments and services work most effectively together with a strong emphasis on quality improvement and value for money (Barker, 2010; Williamson et al., 2010; NIHCE, 2011). Wallen et al. (2010) support this and suggest that EBP can improve the quality of care and outcome for patients, as it fosters a culture in organisations that promotes best practices as opposed to care that is based solely on tradition. An EBP approach also improves practitioners' skills and reduces practice variation and healthcare costs. This evidence base is likely to grow as more evaluative studies are conducted.

Recent years have also seen a rise in litigation in healthcare, resulting in the need for practitioners to be accountable and able to justify their actions (Williamson et al., 2010). Adopting an approach to care that is evidence based supports individual accountability and also assists organisations in justifying their approach to care delivery. As early as 1972, it was suggested that limited healthcare resources should be used effectively for those interventions that have been shown to be effective (Cochrane, 1972). Today, the EBP approach is fundamental to quality improvement strategies, clinical effectiveness and the clinical governance agenda in the NHS. These aspects are returned later and explored in more detail.

Paramedics have begun to embrace EBP more recently, with the move of their initial preparation into higher education (Griffiths and Mooney, 2012) and in these relatively new and emerging fields of practice, there may not be a substantial body of research. Subsequently, there is a need to draw on research carried out in other disciplines to inform care and employ a systematic, structured approach to embracing EBP. This assists in ensuring that evidence transfers appropriately across professions to promote inter-professional learning (Donohoe and Blaber, 2008).

The process and skills required when undertaking evidence based practice

There has been an explosion of available evidence in recent years, much of it available to patients via the internet and they may be more informed than healthcare practitioners about their care. It is challenging but important for busy practitioners to keep up to date with the range and scope of evidence available; nevertheless, practitioners may not have the skills to employ EBP and therefore there is a gap between the best evidence and practice (Hallas and Melnyk, 2003; Shapiro, 2007).

In discussing approaches to EBP and the skills required, it is important to distinguish between the role of practitioners in generating evidence to inform healthcare (which can be used for EBP) and the process by which all practitioners utilise and evaluate this evidence. Not all practitioners will be involved in the generation of evidence to support and underpin care delivery. However, all practitioners should aim to underpin their care delivery with the best available evidence.

The process of EBP is generally identified as having a number of stages, often presented cyclically. The approach to EBP adopted by the JBI is easy to follow if starting out on this process. They identify three simple stages which are

1. access the evidence that is relevant to the field
2. appraise the value of that evidence
3. use that evidence to inform care delivery

These simple steps to EBP can be broken down further and Figure 4.1 presents a composite summary of the key stages. At each stage of the cycle, practitioners need a set of skills to be able to employ EBP and to be able to formulate and clarify the question to be asked and to identify potential evidence sources.

Stage 1: Formulate and clarify the question to be asked

The first consideration for EBP is identifying the area of practice or question that evidence is required to inform. Developing a clear and focused question will make the rest of the process more effective. This will make searching electronic databases more efficient in arriving at the final outcome as it is less likely that there will be a need to go back over the same ground. Initially, a broad area of practice may be identified for investigation, this broad area then needs to be narrowed down to a specific focus.

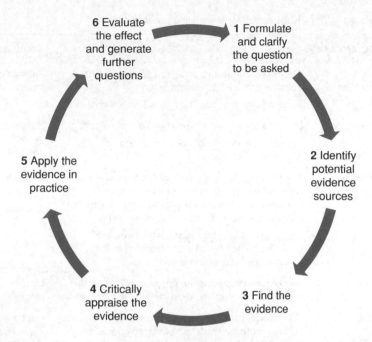

Figure 4.1 The cyclical approach to evidence based practice. Data from Hewitt-Taylor (2003), BMJ (2009), Barker (2010), Williamson et al. (2010) and Joanna Briggs Institute (2010).

Use of the *PICO* acronym (Craig, 2007; Barker, 2010) is recommended to frame appropriate and focused questions. This approach suggests identifying the following:

1. *Problem* (P) for which evidence is sought; for example, patients presenting with symptoms of a myocardial infarct (MI) or the problem of dealing how to handle relatives witnessing resuscitation attempts.
2. *Intervention* (I) to be explored in relation to this patient/problem should be identified; for example, pharmaceutical approaches to pain relief in MI or the legal framework that underpins witnessed resuscitation.
3. *Comparison* (C) intervention may be explored. This is seen as optional and will not apply in every case. If we look at the example related to MI, a search might be conducted for evidence of pharmaceutical and alternative approaches to pain relief in MI.
4. *Outcome* (O) to make a statement about the desired outcome. For the examples given, this could be whether pharmaceutical approaches to pain relief are enhanced by alternative therapies and the potential legal consequences for practitioners of their advice to relatives wishing to witness (or not witness) their relative whilst undergoing resuscitation.

Table 4.1 The PICO process for formulating questions

PICO process		Example
Patient/ population	Start with your patient or patient population and describe their characteristics For example, age, sex and medical conditions	Patients experiencing major trauma
Intervention	Describe the intervention that you are considering For example, drug treatment, dressings and alternative therapies	Hospital patient is taken to lead clinician on arrival in hospital
Comparison	If appropriate, identify what are the alternative approaches that could be used as a comparison to the intervention you are exploring. This may be the current treatment that patients are receiving NB: this point may be omitted where you are exploring patient experiences rather than the effectiveness of an intervention	Consultant or nurse-led care Local accident and emergency or trauma centre
Outcome	Identify what you hope the outcome will be for the patient, what effect you want the intervention to have	Long term cost-effective rehabilitation for patients
Time	Sometimes, it may be appropriate to add a fifth letter 'T' to indicate the time frame over which you are considering the question	Over a 6-month period across the summer months (May–October)

In relation to the examples used, the PICO approach would result in the following questions:

1. What guidance exists for effective pharmaceutical management of pain in patients presenting with MI and can this be supplemented by alternative therapies?
2. What is the legal position that can guide practitioners in deciding how to advise relatives who wish to witness their relative undergoing resuscitation?

This gives a clear focus for identifying an evidence base. Some authors add a *T* to the *PICO* acronym to represent time frame. This is illustrated in Table 4.1 together with clinical examples. Box 4.3 offers additional guidance and support to gain a wider understanding and application of *PICO(T)*. Further examples of the application of the acronym can be found in Craig and Pearson (2007), Ireland (2007), Fitzpatrick (2007b), Centre for Evidence Based Medicine (CEBM) (2009a) and Barker (2010).

Box 4.3 Formulating the right question

Think of a question from your own practice.

Access the CEBM guidance on asking focused questions at http://www.cebm.net/index.aspx?o=1036

And write a PICO(T) question that you could follow up.

Stage 2: Identify potential evidence sources

Once a clear question/focus of investigation has been established, the process moves on to gathering the evidence. There is much debate surrounding what is evidence and whether all evidence is equally valuable. The classic definition of EBM by Sackett et al. (1996) refers to the clinician judging the evidence that is appropriate to use in their field of practice. This is potentially a difficult and time-consuming task, yet an essential skill in implementing EBP.

Within the EBM literature, there is a recognised hierarchy of evidence. Initially, this focused on effectiveness, and therefore randomised control trials (RCTs) featured at the top of most evidence hierarchies. RCTs are quantitative studies that generate numerical data which can be analyzed statistically and are therefore seen as the most rigorous way of assessing the cost effectiveness of a treatment. More recently, systematic reviews are increasingly featuring at the top of hierarchies. They are a compilation of several RCTs and are less likely to be misleading. A typical hierarchy of evidence for quantitative research sources in EBM is presented in Box 4.4.

Box 4.4   Typical hierarchy for quantitative research evidence in EBM

1. Systematic reviews and meta-analyses of RCTs
2. Evidence from one or more well-designed RCTs
3. Evidence from other experimental/quantitative studies
4. Evidence from descriptive/qualitative studies; expert committee reports
5. Expert opinion

Source. Data from Evans (2003) and Barker (2010).

Several authors (Evans, 2003; Rycroft-Malone et al., 2004b; Fitzpatrick, 2007b; Barker 2010; JBI, 2011) suggest that a focus solely on effectiveness misses other dimensions of practice that are equally important in assessing and gathering evidence for practice, notably the potential interaction of research evidence with practitioner and patient variables. Rycroft-Malone et al. (2004b), Barker (2010) and Rolfe (2012) discuss that in order to explore alternative forms of evidence to quantitative research we need to consider the nature of the knowledge that we use to inform care.

We also need to consider the nature of the knowledge that we use to inform care. Broadly, knowledge can be seen as falling into one of two categories, propositional or non-propositional (Barker, 2010). Rolfe (2012) suggests that propositional knowledge is sometimes referred to as theoretical knowledge. This is gained from formal learning settings and generally derived from research (most commonly, quantitative); therefore, it can be generalised across a number of different situations. The other form of knowledge, referred to as non-propositional is informal, implicit and mainly derived through practice (Barker, 2010). Eraut (2000) identifies a number of situations where practitioners may demonstrate this form of knowledge, for example, knowledge that enables the making of rapid, intuitive responses to practice situations and knowledge that is embedded in taken-for-granted activities that are daily engaged. Rolfe (2012) breaks the non-propositional knowledge further into three types used by practitioners:

1. *Knowing how* – practical knowledge gained from simulated or real practice learning.
2. *Knowing why* – the deeper understanding of situations, gained from experience that allows practitioners, for example, to work outside of standard procedures.
3. *Knowing who* – the personal knowledge we gain through experience, of ourselves and our patients/clients that enables the application of knowledge to individual situations.

These non-propositional sources of knowledge that inform our practice may not appear to be useful in generalising across situations and drawing conclusions for use as the basis of EBP due to their personal nature. However, Rycroft-Malone et al. (2004b) suggest that if this knowledge is debated, discussed and verified by practitioners across practice settings, it has the potential to become formal propositional knowledge. This process can take place through practitioners initially reflecting during or after caring for patients on how they made the decisions that they did. Schön (1983) referred to this as reflection in or on action and if a number of reflective accounts across a range of practitioners are analysed in the form of a qualitative research project, they do have the potential to become a reliable source of evidence for EBP.

Rycroft-Malone et al. (2004b) suggest that practitioners need to draw on multiple sources of knowledge which have been informed by a range of critically and publicly scrutinised evidence. The range of evidence sources that practitioners can draw on, other than primary research is clinical experience; patients, clients and carers, informed by the local context and environment; legislation and public health campaigns; case reports and case series and expert opinion.

Harbour and Miller (2001) suggest that a hierarchy of evidence should consider how relevant and applicable the evidence is to the target patient group; the consistency of the evidence base identified, and finally the likely clinical impact of the intervention for which evidence is sought. Rycroft-Malone et al. (2004b) give a succinct summary of the debate surrounding evidence and draw two key conclusions; firstly that evidence needs to be 'independently observed and verified' and secondly that any evidence

Table 4.2   Different classifications of evidence

Research	Clinical audit	Service reviews
Establishes and defines what constitutes best practice	Assess the extent to which care is consistent with best practice and/or achieves expected outcomes	Aim to provide a snapshot description of the state of a service, usually in one locality
Enhances quality by producing knowledge to inform guidelines of best practice		Usually concerned with inputs rather than processes or outcomes

Source: Data from NCAAG (2009b).

used to inform patient care has been subject to scrutiny. Therefore, practitioners should be encouraged to access evidence from formal research where possible (Rolfe, 2012): applying the criteria of critical appraisal to establish the quality of the evidence and drawing on other sources where research may not be available. This may prompt practitioners to identify where further research is required.

Stage 3: Finding the evidence

There is a plethora of evidence that can be used, but the clinical effectiveness agenda for evidence based care in the NHS is seen as being informed by three main types of evidence:

1. research
2. clinical audit
3. service reviews

It is important to identify the key differences between these sources as they are sometimes confused. Table 4.2 offers a brief description of the differences between them.

What is research?

The NHS and National Research Ethics Service (2009) indicate that the primary aim of research is to derive generalisable new knowledge, in order to find out what we should be doing with regard to treatment or the service provided to patients. Quantitative research predominates, particularly RCTs, but other approaches to research may be more relevant to practitioners in some settings.

There are broadly two accepted ways of approaching research, depending on how the person undertaking it views the world, our place in it and relationships between people and other aspects of the world. The first approach is positivism, in which the researcher believes that the world is ordered and regular, knowledge is objective and can therefore be observed, measured and relationships determined. Rolfe (2012) indicates that positivist research aims to avoid any influence from the views and opinions of the researcher. This approach to research is often seen as the most reliable source for EBP. However, this may be difficult to achieve when carrying out research into patient perceptions and experiences of healthcare. Researchers working in the positivist paradigm normally collect *quantitative* data – which can be measured and subjected to statistical tests, for example, RCTs, which are often referred to as the 'gold standard' of evidence sources.

In contrast, the second approach is interpretative research. Researchers working in the interpretative paradigm believe that we each individually construct a view of the world and seek to understand it. This cannot be measured using the objective approach of positivist research, but needs to be explored in depth with each participant to understand their interpretation (Cohen et al., 2011). Rolfe (2012) indicates that those undertaking interpretive research recognise that in the course of collecting research data, there is a connection between the researcher and the participants and that objectivity is therefore not possible. If conducted well, however, they will acknowledge this connection and the possible impact on the findings of the study. Interpretative researchers collect *qualitative data*, which focus on describing meaning and providing a more in-depth and rich description of the situation being studied (Cohen et al., 2011).

Increasingly, healthcare researchers are recognising that there are aspects of both these approaches that can be of benefit as they may require objective data that can be measured numerically (quantitative data) together with explanations that help to explain that data through interviews with patients by which qualitative data will be generated. This is often referred to as mixed method research (Rolfe, 2012), and Cooper et al. (2007, 2011) suggest that this is particularly useful in exploring complex problems. Cooper et al. (2011) devote an entire article to designing mixed method research for emergency care and cite useful examples where this approach has been utilised could add the hierarchy structure.

Clinical audit and service reviews?

There are many similarities between clinical audit and service reviews, as both measure activities within an identified area by drawing on existing data. The key difference is that service reviews take a snapshot view of care and identify the standard of delivery at a given time. In contrast, clinical audit measures care against identified standards and makes recommendations for improving that care where relevant.

The process of clinical audit is a key aspect of quality management and the process is responsible for generating the data on which other activities such as commissioning and regulation of care depend (National Clinical

Table 4.3   Stages in the clinical audit process

Stage 1	Preparing for audit	Set standard
Stage 2	Selecting criteria	Develop audit tool
Stage 3	Measuring level of performance	Collect and interpret data
Stage 4	Making improvements	Take action
Stage 5	Sustaining improvement	Evaluate action and set/refine standard
	NIHCE (2002)	*NHS Scotland (2007)*

Audit Advisory Group (NCAAG), 2009a). Clinical audit can be seen as a five-stage process (see Table 4.3). These stages demonstrate some similarities with the EBP process which include collection and interpretation of evidence, the application of this evidence in practice and identification of new questions/standards to be considered in the following cycle.

Despite these similarities, there are some differences in the two processes. EBP draws on evidence from sources such as research studies to inform questions about practice, which is critically appraised before determining its applicability to the identified situation/question.

The evidence identified through the process of EBP will inform the development and implementation of clinical standards. Clinical audit focuses on comparing what is currently happening in practice with the evidence of best practice, which may be set out in previously identified standards (NHS Scotland, 2007). The implementation of standards is subsequently evaluated through clinical audit. The clinical audit process can draw on a wide range of resources across disciplines and can be carried out at many levels within the organisation, from individual healthcare staff, interdisciplinary or multidisciplinary teams or across whole organisations.

The National Clinical Audit Support Programme (NCASP) (2011) oversees a wide range of audits that looks at the care patients are receiving in a particular field. These give clinicians reliable and valid information to help review their performance and identify areas where they can make improvements. An example of this with particular relevance to emergency care is the information generated by the Myocardial Infarction National Audit Project (MINAP), which is managed by the National Institute for Cardiovascular Outcomes Research (NICOR) at University College London (NICOR, 2011). This was established in 1998, to audit the standard of care delivered to manage myocardial infarctions in ambulance services and NHS hospitals in England and Wales and to measure their performance against national standards (Healthcare Quality Improvement Partnership, 2009; NICOR, 2011). An annual report provides hospitals and ambulance services with a record of their management and compares this with nationally and internationally agreed standards. In addition, the MINAP audit also supports the Care Quality Commission data supplied on their heart surgery website.

The Care Quality Commission is an independent regulator, responsible for monitoring the standard of health and social care services in England, across hospitals, dentists, ambulances, care homes and services in people's own homes. They carry out reviews of services which provide useful information for practitioners to inform their care; these can be accessed on their website at http://www.cqc.org.uk/public/reports-surveys-and-reviews.

A useful source of audit data for emergency practitioners is published by The National Audit Office (NAO) which scrutinises public spending on behalf of parliament, with three strategic priorities:

1. informed government
2. financial management and reporting
3. cost-effective delivery of services

Transforming NHS Ambulance Services (NAO, 2011) explores ambulance trusts to see if they

- Provide a cost-effective service to patients seeking urgent and emergency care.
- Operate in such a way as to minimise costs to the wider health service (i.e. the relationship between the ambulance service and the rest of the NHS).

This report sets out the requirements for a cost-effective ambulance service with some key recommendations including that 'ambulance services need to take more opportunities to learn from each other' and that 'the ability to improve performance is limited by a lack of data on patient outcomes and a lack of comparative information that can be used to benchmark performance' (NAO, 2011, pp. 7–8). These findings have direct relevance and add weight to the agenda for EBP and should further encourage individual practitioners to engage with the skills.

Literature searching

Having established that there are a variety of different sources of evidence for EBP, the principal approach to source this evidence will be via a thorough literature search. This search should use a systematic approach to get the best results and there is guidance for practitioners to develop these essential skills. Beaven and Craig (2007) and Barker (2010) identify key stages in this process and these are summarised in Box 4.5.

Box 4.5   Key stages in conducting a literature search

Generate a word list from your question
Familiarise yourself with common search terms (e.g. Boolean logic; truncation)
Identify the databases and sources available to you
Identify a source of help to assist with your early searches

Electronic databases are the most useful tool for searching the literature and higher education; NHS and public libraries will offer guidance on their use. Also, there may be a need to conduct a hand search through paper-based documents, especially if drawing on some of the 'alternative' sources to research identified above such as policies and procedures and patient information leaflets (Mooney, 2012). The CEBM (2009b) offers a useful exercise for moving from a question formulated (using PICO) to a strategy for searching the literature. A useful approach is to develop a search strategy that identifies the keywords you wish to search for together with alternatives. Also, consideration should be given on any limitations to the search such as how many years to go back, in order to avoid accessing too many articles. Mooney (2012) discusses in more depth a number of factors to be considered in conducting an effective literature search. It is not intended to discuss how to do a literature search in this chapter.

The next stage is that of critical appraisal to enable judgements to be made about the value of the evidence.

Stage 4: Critically appraise the evidence

Critical appraisal is an important step in EBP as we should not assume that all evidence that is available in print or via the internet is 'good' evidence to be used in addressing the question we have set. When appraising the evidence, Burls (2009, p. 1) suggests that critical appraisal is the 'process of systematically appraising the research to assess its reliability and validity, and the value and relevance in a particular context'. Gibson and Glenny (2007) indicate that critical appraisal can be broken down into three elements:

1. Identifying whether the results of the study are valid and of sufficient quality to produce results to inform clinical practice
2. Scrutinising the results and putting them into context for the patient/client group
3. Identifying whether the results will help in the local context and can be applied in the identified clinical setting

Critical appraisal tools

Critical appraisal tools have been developed to facilitate a standard approach to appraising the evidence. Due to the variety of types of evidence now available to practitioners, the tool chosen for appraisal will need to be suitable for that evidence. As quantitative and qualitative research studies adopt a different approach, critical appraisal requires tools that focus on different aspects. Caldwell et al. (2005) presents an appraisal tool that can be applied to both quantitative and qualitative research. This tool provides a good 'entry level' approach where practitioners may be initially unsure of the methodological approach adopted in the selected evidence or where a range of evidence being reviewed adopts both approaches. This encourages practitioners to start by considering the title of the research and if it reflects its contents, the credentials of the authors – are they credible to be writing about this topic area? Following these introductory questions, the tool relates to specific questions about quantitative and qualitative studies. For example, for a quantitative study, it is important to identify whether the experimental hypothesis is clearly stated. For a qualitative study, the context in which the study is being conducted is a key consideration. For both types of study, the population being studied and how they have been selected is an important consideration, but the focus is slightly different in the two approaches.

Having explored the design of quantitative and qualitative studies separately, this tool then identifies three key questions to be asked about all studies being evaluated, these relate to the presentation of results; the quality of the discussion and of the conclusion. Critical appraisal of quantitative studies focuses on the validity and reliability of a study, for instance, does it measure what it claims to be measuring, are the measurements consistent and if repeated would they get the same results (Barker, 2010). Qualitative studies, on the other hand, should be judged by whether the methods used are credible, and dependable, whether they can be confirmed by other sources and transferred to other situations (Caldwell et al., 2005).

One of the most often used tools for critical appraisal is the Solutions for Public Health Critical Appraisal Skills website (www.sph.nhs.uk) which provides a variety of appraisal tools for different types of evidence, for example, systematic reviews, RCTs, and qualitative studies together with other specifically targeted study types (NHS Solutions for Public Health, 2010). Barker (2010) also includes, as appendices to her book, useful examples of critical appraisal tools with clearly structured questions. Practitioners inexperienced in the use of critical appraisal tools will benefit from working with someone who has the experience of using the tools to gain confidence to make valid judgements about the benefit of the studies in their practice environment.

Healthcare professionals will not only access evidence from research studies, but also from other sources such as clinical guidelines and protocols (these are discussed under stage 5: applying the evidence). The skills involved in critical appraisal of these documents are essentially the same as already discussed; however, due the purpose and structure of the documents, different questions will be asked.

Sanderlin and AbdulRahim (2007) present a useful article discussing the particular factors to consider when appraising these documents, presenting a question-based appraisal tool. For example, they suggest that questions should be asked about the make-up and expertise of the panel who prepared the guideline; the strength of the data evidence used to prepare the guideline and whether it takes into account what is acceptable and practical for that particular patient group. In addition, the Appraisal of Guidelines and Research Evaluation Collaboration (2001) have developed a tool for appraising clinical guidelines, which asks a series of 24 questions about relating to the purpose of the guideline, stakeholder involvement in its development, concluding with a question as to whether the guideline should be recommended for use in practice. The tool is designed to be used by policy makers, guideline developers, healthcare providers and educators. It is recommended that a minimum of two appraisers (but preferably four) work on each appraisal and this may offer opportunities for those less experienced to work with experienced appraisers.

Evans (2003) suggests that by widening out the criteria for evaluating evidence through the inclusion of other factors, evidence sources other than RCTs can be deemed valuable. He cites as examples the feasibility of care interventions – are they practical to implement in physical, cultural or financial terms. Secondly, whether the interventions are appropriate for the context in which they will be used and how are they likely to be experienced by individuals, for example, a particular religious group.

Having carried out an appraisal of the evidence relating to the identified question, practitioners move onto the next stage and face a challenge to implement their findings in practice.

Stage 5: Apply the evidence in practice

Gathering evidence to support practice and being aware of tools such as clinical guidelines and protocols will only impact on care if these are shared with colleagues and implemented in practice. Patients will only benefit from efforts to seek out appropriate and relevant evidence if this results in changes to practice where appropriate. Barker (2010) describes the process of transferring evidence into practice as daunting, difficult and complex as it is not just a case of informing people about up-to-date research findings. Knowing the best evidence does not mean that this will automatically filter into practice. Clinical guidelines and protocols may be an approach/strategy that may be successful in implementing evidence in practice.

Clinical guidelines and protocols

Evidence generated by the processes of research, clinical and service review informs practice through the production of clinical guidelines and protocols. Clinical guidelines have been available to practitioners to inform care for a number of years. The Scottish Intercollegiate Guidelines Network (SIGN) began producing clinical guidelines in 1993, whilst the National Institute for Health and Clinical Excellence (NIHCE) has been producing guidelines since its inception in 1999. With the increasing emphasis on clinical effectiveness, however, they have more recently developed a higher profile.

What are clinical guidelines?

The RCN (2009) suggests that motivating factors for the development of clinical guidelines have been unacceptable variations in practice patterns; concern with appropriateness of care and increasing healthcare costs. Many organisation agencies commission and develop clinical guidelines at national level (see Box 4.6). Clinical guidelines are defined by NIHCE (2011) as

> recommendations on the appropriate treatment and care of people with specific diseases and conditions . . . based on the best available evidence.

Box 4.6   Organisations that commission and develop clinical guidelines

National Institute for Health and Clinical Evidence – http://www.nice. org.uk/

National Clinical Guideline Centre – http://www.ncgc.ac.uk/

Guidelines and Audit Implementation Network – http://www.gain-ni.org/

Scottish Intercollegiate Guidelines Network (SIGN) – http://www.sign. ac.uk/

It is important to consider that although guidelines are based on best-available evidence for specific diseases and conditions, it is important to note that research will exclude certain groups such as children, the elderly above a certain age, patients with a range of co-morbidity conditions, so it is important to be mindful that when using the guideline, it may not be appropriate for some patient groups. An example of this will be the Ottawa ankle rules (Stiell et al., 1992) which is a guideline for clinicians in deciding if a patient with a foot and/or ankle injury should be offered an X-ray. The introduction of this guideline significantly reduced the number of patients being X-rayed, thus reducing the cost, time and health risks caused by unnecessary X-rays. The research supporting these guidelines only included participants aged between 16 and 55 years. Therefore, for those patients who are outside of this age range, the Ottawa guidelines would not be able to be applied.

Clinical guidelines should be valid and represent the interests of key groups and clearly define the patient populations that they affect. In addition, they should be developed using language that is readily understood by all and flexible in terms of their expectations. Finally, a review date should be set and they should be able to be readily translated into clinical audit criteria.

NIHCE (2011) suggest that clinical guidelines help healthcare professionals in their work to support decision making. In most cases, guidelines will be adhered to but you must remember that they are advisory and not sub-stitute for knowledge and skills as there will be circumstances where your knowledge and skills will override them. As a registered professional, it is a requirement that you keep your knowledge and skills up to date and use appropriate up-to-date evidence (NMC, 2008; HCPC, 2012). Also, you need to consider that not all guidelines may be up to date, may not include all the information required to support your decision making or may not re-flect individual situation. Sometimes, the accuracy, reliability and currency of the guideline may be apparent, as contemporary evidence will super-sede these. Subsequently, individuals using these guidelines must ensure that they have the appropriate knowledge and skills to enable appropri-ate interpretation and they should be aware of these new innovations or alterations after the date of publication may not be included.

Advantages and disadvantages of clinical guidelines

There are many potential advantages of the use of clinical guidelines to inform care. The RCN (2009) suggests that a guideline will assist decision-makers in changing the process of healthcare to improve outcomes for pa-tients, ensure efficient use of healthcare resources and reduce variations to practice. Although it has been shown in rigorous evaluations that clini-cal practice guidelines can improve the quality of care, SIGN (2008) warn that local ownership of the implementation process is crucial to success in changing practice. Woolf et al. (1999) identified the potential benefits and limitations of clinical guidelines under three clear headings: those for pa-tients, for healthcare professionals and for healthcare systems.

What are clinical protocols?

In contrast to clinical guidelines, protocols are a specific framework with specific criteria for providing an aspect of patient care (RCN, 2009). Proto-cols are sometimes used interchangeably with clinical guidelines but key differences are that protocols are usually developed at local level to im-plement national standards, specify the treatment that is endorsed by the employer, vary in the degree to which they are optional for practitioners and may not be evidence based.

Examples of protocols include patient group directions (PGDs), which provide step-by-step descriptions of care. For further information on PGDs, see Chapter 8.

How we use evidence in practice

Implementing change to practice based on the evidence base can take place at a number of levels. This can range from changing personal practice or that of the immediate team to changes that have a national or international impact (Barker, 2010). Initially, practitioners are likely to be involved principally in individual or team-level change. In order to make use of evidence in practice, time is needed for thorough consideration of the change, an awareness of the change management process and access to support at various levels in the organisation.

Planning for a change in practice

Having identified a recommendation from the evidence for implementation in practice, use can be made of the principles for promoting change in an organisation. The first stage in implementing a change is careful preparation for that change and factors that need be taken into consideration are whether an individual has control over the proposed change (i.e. impact on the multidisciplinary team); whether it is within their sphere of practice; whether there are any resource implications and whether those involved have the education and skills to facilitate change or will there be a requirement for the team to develop new skills (Fitzpatrick, 2007c).

Rycroft-Malone (2004) indicates that the context in which we try to implement change is crucial and key success factors are that individuals feel valued, the necessary resources are available and teamwork practices are effective, before embarking on the change.

As part of the planning process, it is beneficial to identify any barriers that might exist to the change being successful and also to identify the 'gap' between current practice and where we would like to be after the change has occurred (Barker, 2010). Good use can be made of tools to analyse a proposed change, for example, a SWOT analysis (see Box 4.7) or simply by asking:

- *How* can the team be encouraged to embrace the proposed change?
- *What* should the change achieve and what will indicate success? and finally
- *Why* is there a need for change from the existing approach to the planned change?

(Barker, 2010)

Identifying barriers to using EBP in advance can allow for anticipation of ways to overcome these as part of the implementation of the change.

Implementing a change

Having considered factors that may impact on planning the change, implementation requires a clear set of goals to be achieved, a timeline and an implementation strategy. There are many suggestions for factors that will make a change happen more effectively and be sustained (see Box 4.8).

> **Box 4.7   A SWOT analysis for proposed change**
>
> **Strengths:**
> What are my strengths in relation to the proposed change?
> What skills do I have that can help the change happen?
> What are the potential positive consequences of this change for the organisation?
>
> **Weaknesses:**
> What are my limitations in relation to the proposed change?
> What skills do I need to develop to facilitate the change?
> What are the potential negative consequences of this change for the organisation?
>
> **Opportunities:**
> What opportunities are there for me to gain the skills I need?
> What resources and support are available in the organisation to help me?
> What longer-term opportunities could the change open up for the team?
>
> **Threats:**
> What barriers are there to making the change happen?
> What longer-term threats could the change result in for the team?

Rycroft-Malone (2004) suggests that this can be framed under three key headings:

- The quality of the evidence and the variety of sources that it is drawn from
- The context in which the change is taking place
- The quality of the available facilitation in helping the change to happen

These can be ranked from high to low to identify aspects likely to affect the success of implementing change based on the evidence.

Barriers to using evidence based practice

There are many areas of practice in healthcare that are not based on current evidence for a number of reasons (Hallas and Melnyk, 2003; Rycroft-Malone et al., 2004a; MacGuire, 2006; Barker, 2010). Firstly, practitioners may lack awareness of the available evidence or doubt its value and credibility. In some cases, appropriate and relevant evidence may not be available in their field. They may oppose EBP because they perceive that only evidence from RCTs can be recognised. Practitioners may be overwhelmed

> **Box 4.8   Factors that can influence effective change in practice**
>
> Support at all levels of the organisation
> Clear evidence of the benefits of the change
> Sufficient resources to sustain any changes made
> Identifying 'champions' who are committed to the change and will pro-
> mote it amongst colleagues, e.g. provide a database of people in the
> organisation with practical knowledge of change management, to en-
> courage networking and learning
> Ensuring effective relationships between all members of the multidisci-
> plinary team that the change impacts on, e.g. multidisciplinary discussion
> forums
> Everyone feels involved and some ownership of the process
> Providing skills in, for example, action research, basic statistics and how
> to analyse and display them and for constructing project management
> network diagrams
>
> Data from Iles and Sutherland (2001), Rycroft-Malone (2004), and
> Barker (2010).

by the volume of information available; where evidence is available, it may
be some time before it filters down to practitioners and is implemented.
Practitioners may also lack the time and/or skills to critically appraise evidence. As a result, they prefer to leave this to those who they see more
effectively equipped to do this such as those in specialist posts. Finally,
they may lack support from their organisation to explore and implement
up-to-date evidence. Other factors such as the management system, available resources and patient/carer perceptions of change may also obstruct
the implementation of EBP (Barker, 2010).

Stage 6: Evaluate the effect and generate further questions

The final stage of the EBP cycle is planning for evaluation of change, to
identify what impact it has had and identify whether further change is
needed. Evaluation can establish whether the original objectives and benefits of change have been achieved and can also lead to further questions
about practice. In this way, the need for further change may become apparent but the process of evaluating change may also contribute further
to the evidence base in that field (Rycroft-Malone, 2004). The framework
used to evaluate change needs to capture the complexity of the organisation and of the stakeholders involved in the change – for example, members of the multidisciplinary team, patients and clients and relatives. It will
therefore be more effective if it draws on broad and multiple sources of

evidence (Guba and Lincoln, 1989). Any evaluation that involves gathering data from staff, patients, relatives or carers should gain ethical approval in the same way as conducting a research project.

Contributing to the evidence base

As questions are formulated to investigate from existing practice and evidence is accessed to answer these questions, further areas for investigation will inevitably be raised; or areas identified that are poorly researched. Ideas may be generated for improving the quality of healthcare delivery by the team and this may motivate individuals to gather evidence about this with a view to improving effectiveness. Alternatively, a 'gap' may be identified where there is evidence of best practice but clinical guidelines do not exist to inform and sustain this best practice. This may provide opportunities to work with colleagues in researching these areas or developing new clinical guidelines, thus adding to the evidence base.

Practitioners may have opportunities to become involved in research projects, in conjunction with researchers in their organisation. Griffiths and Mooney (2012) suggest that in developing professions such as paramedic practice, a key challenge is for more practitioners to become leaders of research projects that can inform the evidence base.

There are also a number of resources available to guide practitioners in preparing clinical guidelines. Initially, it is good practice to establish whether there is someone identified in the organisation that has responsibility for EBP or research and development as they will be able to assist in the process of guideline development. Broughton and Rathbone (2001) outline the features of a good clinical guideline and suggest that for clinical guidelines to be successful, they should be developed and implemented with the involvement of clinicians, providers, purchasers and the public. They provide a useful checklist for evaluating guidelines as they are developed. Support for promoting EBP and adding to the evidence base can be sought from professional organisations and charities, for example, the Health Foundation offer funding and support to teams for this type of work (http://www.health.org.uk/areas-of-work/programmes/shine-twelve/).

Professional standards in relation to evidence based practice

Practitioners registered with either the Health and Care Professions Council (HCPC) or the Nursing and Midwifery Council (NMC) are required as part of their *Standards of Conduct, Performance and Ethics* to demonstrate that they keep their professional knowledge and skills up to date and act within the limits of their knowledge, skills and experience (NMC, 2008; HCPC, 2012). In addition, the NMC (2008) add a requirement to use the best available evidence to inform the care that practitioners deliver. Key factors that are highlighted by these standards are firstly that the knowledge that underpins practice must be of a good quality, up to date and relevant to the situation that the practitioner is working in. This includes the delivery of care and recommendation of products or services. Secondly, for both professional bodies, this requirement is linked to continued registration, which emphasises the importance of EBP to individual practitioners. The NMC (2008) stress the importance of practitioners sharing their skills and experience with colleagues and taking advice from them when required. In addition, it is important to share and disseminate knowledge as this is important to applying the evidence. Practitioners need to be aware that, although very rare, each year a small number of healthcare practitioners are suspended or removed from their register as a result of incidents that can be directly traced to the quality of the knowledge base and evidence underpinning their care, examples of such cases can be found on the NMC and HPC websites http://www.nmc-uk.org/Hearings/Hearings-and-outcomes/ and http://www.hpc-uk.org/complaints/. These can form the basis of discussion in teams about their responsibilities for promoting EBP. Box 4.9 illustrates this cycle for EBP and how this can be applied to practice.

Box 4.9   Illustration to summarise the approach to evidence based practice

Formulate and clarify the question to be asked:
Using the PICO(T) acronym, a team working in the Emergency Department have devised the following question:
'What is the legal position that can guide practitioners in deciding how to advise relatives who wish to witness their relative undergoing resuscitation?'

Identify potential evidence sources and find the evidence:
Appropriate evidence is sourced from a literature search, for which guidance is sought from the librarian in the hospital library. A key document forms a starting point for the search, providing a useful summary of the position surrounding witnessed resuscitation:
Resuscitation Council UK (1996) – Resuscitation Council guidance on witnessed resuscitation.
A systematic review – often considered the 'gold standard' of evidence is accessed.
Scott Dingeman et al. (2007) – this explores the position with regard to parents witnessing resuscitation of children.

Together with a range of research studies, both quantitative and qualitative including:

Gordon et al. (2011) – which is a descriptive study exploring doctor's attitudes to witnessed resuscitation

Booth et al. (2004) – which uses a survey approach to exploring witnessed resuscitation in UK emergency departments.

A range of other literature including clinical guidelines and protocols are sourced (both at national and local Trust level) including RCN (2002) and Reynolds et al. (2007).

This illustrates the shift in emphasis over recent years from sole reliance on RCTs and systematic reviews for EBP.

Critically appraise the evidence:

A range of appraisal tools are used, with guidance from the Trust research department who work with the team to sift the evidence for the robustness of each article/document and the appropriateness to their clinical situation.

This leads to a conclusion that current practice in the department is largely appropriate and evidence based, but that not all staff are aware of the legal background and therefore their responsibilities to relatives who request to witness resuscitation in the department.

Apply the evidence in practice:

The team works with the Trust research department and representatives from all professional disciplines in the emergency department to draw up a clinical guideline to inform practice around witnessed resuscitation. Guidance on drawing up this guideline is taken from Broughton and Rathbone (2001).

The guideline is then submitted for ratification by the Trust before implementation.

Implementation of the guideline is supported by education sessions for all staff, and this is advertised via the Departmental noticeboard and an email to all staff members. The team also plan for an evaluation of the implementation of the guideline, which includes seeking ethical approval to send a questionnaire to staff and relatives.

Evaluate the effect and generate further questions:

Three months after the implementation of the new guideline, a questionnaire is sent electronically to all staff to canvass their awareness and understanding of it. The relatives of patients who are resuscitated in the department are asked whether they are prepared to complete a questionnaire regarding their experiences, to inform any future changes to the guideline.

Conclusion

McKenna et al. (2000) suggest that there are five commonly held myths about EBP:

- EBP automatically takes patient outcomes into account.
- EBP is the same as clinical effectiveness.
- EBP is the same as research-based practice.
- All evidence in nursing should be research based.
- EBP should always be the desired option.

Some of these have been explored in this chapter and will enable practitioners to have a more informed view about these myths but there are questions that remain to be explored regarding the extent to which individual practitioners can embrace EBP in their everyday practice. However, what cannot be questioned is that all practitioners need to be aware of the EBP agenda and strive to use the best available evidence whenever possible. Furthermore, when faced with a care situation that has not been encountered before, practitioners must demonstrate that they have taken every possible step to seek out and apply the best available evidence to that situation.

References

Appraisal of Guidelines and Research Evaluation Collaboration (2001) *Appraisal of Guidelines Research & Evaluation (AGREE) Instrument.* Available at http://www.agreecollaboration.org/instrument/ (accessed April 2012).

Barker, J. (2010) *Evidence-Based Practice for Nurses.* Sage Publications, London.

Beaven, O. & Craig, J.V. (2007) Searching the literature. In: *Evidence-Based Practice Manual for Nurses*, 2nd edn (eds J.V. Craig & R.L. Smyth). Churchill Livingstone, Edinburgh.

BMJ Evidence Centre (2009) *Building Evidence into Practice.* Available at http://group.bmj.com/products/evidence-centre (accessed January 2012).

Booth, M.G., Woolrich, L. & Kinsella, J. (2004) Family witnessed resuscitation in UK emergency departments: a survey of practice. *European Journal of Anaesthesiology*, **21**, 725–728.

Broughton, R. & Rathbone, B. (2001) *What Makes a Good Clinical Guideline?* Hayward Medical Communications, Kent. Available at http://www.medicine. ox.ac.uk/bandolier/painres/download/whatis/whatareclinguide.pdf (accessed June 2012).

Burls, A. (2009) *What Is Critical Appraisal?* Hayward Medical Communications, Kent. Available at http://www.whatisseries.co.uk/whatis/pdfs/What_is_ crit_appr.pdf (accessed December 2011).

Caldwell, K., Henshaw, L. & Taylor, G. (2005) Developing a framework for critiquing health research. *Journal of Health, Social and Environmental Issues*, **6**(1), 45–53.

Centre for Evidence-Based Medicine (CEBM) (2009a) *Asking Focused Questions*. Available at http://www.cebm.net/index.aspx?o=1036 (accessed March 2012).

Centre for Evidence-Based Medicine (CEBM) (2009b) *Searching Warm-up Exercise*. Available at http://www.cebm.net/index.aspx?o=2311 (accessed March 2012).

Cochrane, A.L. (1972) *Effectiveness and Efficiency. Random Reflections on Health Services*. Nuffield Provincial Hospitals Trust, London.

Cochrane, A.L. (1979) 1931–1971: a critical review with particular reference to the medical profession. In: *Medicines for the Year 2000*, (eds Feeling-Smith, G. & Wells, N.), pp. 1–11. Office of Health Economics, London.

Cohen, L., Manion, L. & Morrison, K. (2011) *Research Methods in Education*. Routledge, Abingdon.

Cooper, S. & Endacott, R. (2007) Generic qualitative research: a design for qualitative research in emergency care? *Emergency Medicine Journal*, **24**(12), 816–819.

Cooper, S., Porter, J. & Endacott, R. (2011) Mixed methods research: a design for emergency care research? *Emergency Medicine Journal*, **28**(8), 682–685.

Craig, J.V. (2007) How to ask the right question. In: *Evidence-Based Practice Manual for Nurses*, 2nd edn (eds J.V. Craig & R.L. Smyth). Churchill Livingstone, Edinburgh.

Craig, J.V. & Pearson, M. (2007) Evidence-based practice in nursing. In: *Evidence-Based Practice Manual for Nurses*, 2nd edn (eds J.V. Craig & R.L. Smyth). Churchill Livingstone, Edinburgh.

Donohoe, R., & Blaber, A. (2008) Professional issues affecting practice. In: *Foundations for Paramedic Practice – A Theoretical Perspective* (ed. A. Blaber). Open University Press, Maidenhead.

Eraut, M. (2000) Non-formal learning and tacit knowledge in professional work. *British Journal of Educational Psychology*, **70**, 113–136.

Evans, D. (2003) Hierarchy of evidence: a framework for ranking evidence evaluating healthcare interventions. *Journal of Clinical Nursing*, **12**, 77–84.

Fitzpatrick, J. (2007a) Finding the research for evidence-based practice – part one – the development of EBP. *Nursing Times*, **103**(17), 32–33.

Fitzpatrick, J. (2007b) Finding the research for evidence-based practice – part two – selecting credible evidence. *Nursing Times*, **103**(18), 32–33.

Fitzpatrick, J. (2007c) Finding the research for evidence-based practice – part three – making a case. *Nursing Times*, **103**(19), 32–33.

Gibson, F. & Glenny, A. (2007) Critical appraisal of quantitative studies 1: is the quality of the study good enough for you to use the findings? In: *Evidence-Based Practice Manual for Nurses*, 2nd edn (eds J.V. Craig & R.L. Smyth). Churchill Livingstone, Edinburgh.

Gordon, E.D., Kramer, E., Couper, I. & Brysiewicz, P. (2011) Family-witnessed resuscitation in emergency departments: doctors' attitudes and practices. *South African Medical Journal*, **101**(10), 765–767.

Griffiths, P. & Mooney, G.P. (2012) Research and the paramedic. In: *The Paramedics Guide to Research. An Introduction* (eds P. Griffiths & G.P. Mooney). Open University Press, Maidenhead.

Guba, E. & Lincoln, Y. (1989) *Fourth Generation Evaluation*. Sage, Beverly Hills.

Hallas, D. & Melnyk, B.M. (2003) Evidence-based practice: the paradigm shift. *Journal of Pediatric Health Care*, **17**(1), 46–49.

Harbour, R. & Miller, J. (2001) A new system for grading recommendations in evidence based guidelines. *British Medical Journal*, **323**(7308), 334.

Health and Care Professions Council (HCPC) (2012) *Standards of Conduct, Performance and Ethics*. Health and Care Professions Council, London.

Healthcare Quality Improvement Partnership Ltd (2009) *Clinical Audit Knowledge Exchange*. Available at http://www.hqip.org.uk/clinical-audit-knowledge-exchange-cake/ (accessed June 2012).

Hewitt-Taylor, J. (2003) Reviewing evidence. *Intensive and Critical Care Nursing*, **19**, 43–49.

Iles, V. & Sutherland, K. (2001) *Organisational Change. A Review for Health Care Managers, Professionals and Researchers*. National Co-ordinating Centre for NHS Service Delivery and Organisation, London. Available at http://www.sdo.nihr.ac.uk/files/adhoc/change-management-review.pdf (accessed April 2012).

Ingersoll, G.L. (2000) Evidence-based nursing: what it is and what it isn't. *Nursing Outlook*, **48**, 151–152.

Ireland, L. (2007) Evidence-based practice. In: *Principles of Professional Studies in Nursing* (eds J. Brown & P. Libberton). Palgrave Macmillan, Basingstoke.

MacGuire, J.M. (2006) Putting nursing research findings into practice: research utilization as an aspect of the management of change. *Journal of Advanced Nursing*, **53**(1), 65–74.

McKenna, H., Cutliffe, J. & McKenna, P. (2000) Evidence-based practice: demolishing some myths. *Nursing Standard*, **14**(16), 39–42.

Mooney, G.P. (2012) Conducting a critical literature review in paramedic practice. In: *The Paramedics Guide to Research. An Introduction* (eds P. Griffiths & G.P. Mooney). Open University Press, Maidenhead.

Muir Gray, J.A. (1997) *Evidence –Based Healthcare*. Churchill Livingstone, New York.

National Audit Office (NAO) (2011) *Transforming NHS Ambulance Services*. Available at http://www.nao.org.uk/default.aspx (accessed December 2011).

National Clinical Audit Advisory Group (NCAAG) (2009a) *What Is Clinical Audit?* Available at http://www.dh.gov.uk/prod_consum_dh/groups/dh_digitalassets/@dh/@en/@ps/@sta/@perf/documents/digitalasset/dh_107462.pdf (accessed July 2011).

National Clinical Audit Advisory Group (NCAAG) (2009b) *About NCAAG*. Available at http://www.dh.gov.uk/ab/NCAAG/DH_097446 (accessed July 2011).

National Clinical Audit Support Programme (NCASP) (2011) *More About the Audits*. Available at http://www.ic.nhs.uk/services/national-clinical-audit-support-programme-ncasp/more-about-the-audits (accessed June 2012).

National Institute for Cardiovascular Outcomes Research (NICOR) (2011) *NICOR*. Available at http://www.ucl.ac.uk/nicor/ (accessed April 2012).

National Institute for Health and Clinical Excellence (NIHCE) (2002) *Principles for Best Practice in Clinical Audit*. Radcliffe Medical Press Ltd, Abingdon.

National Institute for Health and Clinical Excellence (NIHCE) (2011) *Clinical Guidelines*. Available at http://guidance.nice.org.uk/CG (accessed April 2012).

National Research Ethics Service (2009) *Defining Research*. National Patient Safety Agency, London. Available at http://www.nres.npsa.nhs.uk/applications/is-your-project-research/ (accessed April 2012).

NHS Scotland (2007) *Clinical Audit*. Available at http://www.clinical governance.scot.nhs.uk/section2/audit.asp (accessed September 2011).

NHS Solutions for Public Health (2010) *Critical Appraisal Skills Programme*. Available at http://www.sph.nhs.uk/what-we-do/public-health-workforce/resources/critical-appraisals-skills-programme (accessed June 2012).

Nursing and Midwifery Council (NMC) (2008) *The Code: Standards of Conduct, Performance and Ethics for Nurses and Midwives*. NMC, London.

Resuscitation Council UK (1996) *Should Relatives Witness Resuscitation?* Resuscitation Council UK, London.

Reynolds, F., McVittie, P. & Cope, H. (2007) *Resuscitation Policy*. Birmingham Children's Hospital NHS Foundation Trust, Birmingham.

Robertson-Malt, S. (2010) Cochrane corner: advanced trauma life support training for hospital staff. *American Journal of Nursing*, **110**(5), 27.

Rolfe, G. (2012) Knowledge to underpin paramedic practice. In: *The Paramedics Guide to Research. An Introduction* (eds P. Griffiths & G.P. Mooney). Open University Press, Maidenhead.

Royal College of Nursing (RCN) (2002) *Witnessing Resuscitation: Guidance for Nursing Staff*. RCN, London.

Royal College of Nursing (RCN) (2003) *Clinical Governance: An RCN Resource Guide*. RCN, London.

Royal College of Nursing (RCN) (2009) *More About Clinical Guidelines*. Available at http://www.rcn.org.uk/development/practice/clinicalguidelines/more_about_clinical_guidelines (accessed June 2012).

Rycroft-Malone, J. (2004) The PARIHS framework – a framework for guiding the implementation of evidence-based practice. *Journal of Nursing Care Quality*, **19**(4), 297–304.

Rycroft-Malone, J., Harvey, G., Seers, K., Kitson, A., McCormack, B. & Titchen, A. (2004a) An exploration of the factors that influence the implementation of evidence into practice. *Issues in Clinical Nursing*, **13**, 913–924.

Rycroft-Malone, J., Seers, K., Titchen, A., Harvey, G., Kitson, A. & McCormack, B. (2004b) What counts as evidence in evidence-based practice? *Journal of Advanced Nursing*, **47**(1), 81–90.

Sackett, D.L., Rosenberg, W.M.C., Gray, J.A.M., Haynes, R.B. & Richardson, W.S. (1996) Evidence based medicine: what it is and what it isn't. *British Medical Journal*, **312**, 71–72.

Sanderlin, B.W. & AbdulRahim, N. (2007) Evidence-based medicine, Part 6. An introduction to critical appraisal of clinical practice guidelines. *Journal of the American Osteopath Association*, **107**, 321–324.

Schön, D. (1983) *The Reflective Practitioner*. Temple Smith, London.

Scott Dingeman, R., Mitchell, A., Meyer, E.C. & Curley, M.A.Q. (2007) Parent presence during complex invasive procedures and cardiopulmonary resuscitation: a systematic review of the literature. *Pediatrics*, **120**(4), 842–854.

Scottish Intercollegiate Guidelines Network (SIGN) (2008) *SIGN 50 A Guideline Developer's Handbook.* SIGN, Edinburgh. Available at http://www.sign.ac.uk/pdf/sign50.pdf (accessed January 2012).

Shapiro, S.E. (2007) Evidence-based practice for advanced practice emergency nurses. *Advanced Emergency Nursing Journal*, **29**(4), 331–338.

Stiell, I.G., Greenberg, G.H., McKnight, R.D., Nair, R.C., McDowell, I. & Worthington, J.R. (1992) A study to develop clinical decision rules for the use of radiography in acute ankle injuries. *Annuls of Emergency Medicine*, **21**(4), 384–390.

The Joanna Briggs Institute (JBI) (2011) Joanna Briggs Institute. The University of Adelaide. About us. Available at http://www.joannabriggs.edu.au/About%20Us (accessed January 2012).

Wallen, G.R., Mitchell, S.A., Melnyk, B., et al. (2010) Implementing evidence-based practice: effectiveness of a structured multifaceted mentorship programme. *Journal of Advanced Nursing*, **66**(12), 2761–2771.

Williamson, G.R., Jenkinson, T. & Proctor-Childs, T. (2010) *Contexts of Contemporary Nursing*, 2nd edn. Learning Matters, Exeter.

Woolf, S.H., Grol, R., Hutchinson, A., Eccles, M. & Grimshaw, J. (1999) Potential benefits, limitations and harms of clinical guidelines. *British Medical Journal*, **318**, 527–530.

5 Reflection and Reflective Practice

Kay Norman and Val Nixon

Faculty of Health Sciences, Staffordshire University, Stafford, UK

Introduction

Reflection and reflective practice are now seen as core to professional development in many health professions, encouraging a continuous learning approach involving knowledge acquisition and practice improvement (Williams, 2001). Within your role as a healthcare student and registered healthcare practitioner, reflection can lead to an enhanced understanding of the everyday situations you encounter and the issues involved, in order to critically evaluate not only your role in these situations, but also the role of the wider healthcare arena and associated influences, linking theory to practice. This encourages analysis of the issues involved and may include varying methods of reflective practice such as reflective writing, group discussions, peer support, clinical supervision, problem based learning (PBL) and action learning.

Reflection has its roots within philosophical and educational theory which has been discussed and debated for many years (Dewey, 1933; Habermas, 1972). Subsequently, reflection within professional practice related reflection to the scientific theory that professionals make decisions through 'technical rationality' (Schön, 1991, p. 21). This being where professional's knowledge is used to inform their actions within everyday situations and encounters.

As you read further around the concept of reflection, you may come across more recent literature which suggests that reflection has been distorted to suit health professionals and their regulatory bodies, with reflective writing seen as a requirement rather than a concept to embrace (Jarvis, 1992; Hannigan, 2001). However, reflection can be an enlightening process once understood and developed. Within your learning journey, it is important that you take the opportunity to immerse yourself in this process,

Professional Practice in Paramedic, Emergency and Urgent Care, First Edition. Edited by Val Nixon.
© 2013 John Wiley & Sons, Ltd. Published 2013 by John Wiley & Sons, Ltd.

which will encourage increased self-awareness and lead to the development of ideas, critical thinking of varying practice situations, and improvement of practice.

In order to embrace reflective practice, you must be open minded to new ways of thinking and viewing situations, ready to challenge the status quo and previously held assumptions and be self-motivated to continually improve your personal and professional practice and that of your profession. This can lead to an increased self-confidence in questioning custom and practice, new knowledge and understanding and further insight into your own area of skills and attitudes (Teekman, 2000).

This chapter will explore reflection in its various constructs and the variety of ways that it can be utilised within your professional practice, discussing the nature and function of reflection and the associated learning complexities. Definitions of reflection and the concept of reflective practice will be explored to increase your understanding of how this can be incorporated into your practice. There are a variety of methods to support reflective practice and it is beyond the scope of this chapter to explore and analyse these in depth. A brief introduction of group reflection, clinical supervision, PBL and action learning will be offered to demonstrate how these can be utilised and applied to your educational and practice environment. Models of reflection will also be discussed and how these can help you structure your thoughts and subsequent reflective writing. Utilising Gibbs' (1988) model of reflection, an example of a reflective writing offers a critical analysis of a clinical skill procedure. This will demonstrate how reflective practice promotes links between theory and practice.

What is reflection?

- What do we mean by reflection and reflective practice?
- Is it just thinking about my actions?
- Is it a tool just to look backwards?
- Is it focused purely on situations that did not go well?

Take a minute to think about how many times you 'reflect'. We all reflect on a daily basis although it may not be in an academic sense or to the extent that we critically analyse our actions in depth. You may reflect on your way to work about the previous day, your morning so far, conversations you have had, planning what needs to be done, a previous situation that has been on your mind where you 'play it back' thinking was it good/bad, deliberating alternative strategies that could have been adopted in that situation. This can be seen as informal reflection and is a human trait that we all possess, relating to the nature of knowledge and knowledge acquisition which Plato proposed over 2000 years ago (Rolfe et al., 2001).

There are many definitions of reflection depending on the context in which it is being discussed. The obvious thinking of many when hearing the word reflection would be 'reflection in a mirror' which is essentially the simplest way of looking at reflection – looking back at oneself. This is reinforced within the study by Gustafsson and Fagerberg (2004), where nurses described reflection both as an individual activity looking back at their own practice and as 'mirroring', where team members reflected together to exchange ideas and develop care. Over recent years, reflection and reflective practice has developed much further with a multiple of meanings within healthcare professions, with discourses asserting the benefits of reflection in promoting personal development and professional competence (Gilbert, 2001).

Examples of reflection definitions are as follows:

active, persistent and careful consideration of any belief or supposed form of knowledge in the light of the grounds that support it and the further conclusion to which it tends. (Dewey, 1933, p. 118)

the process of internally examining and exploring an issue of concern, triggered by an experience, which creates and clarifies meaning in terms of self, and which results in a changed conceptual perspective. (Boyd and Fayles, 1983, p. 100)

a process of reviewing an experience of practice in order to describe, analyse, evaluate and so inform learning in practice. (Reid, 1993, p. 305)

a form of mental processing with a purpose and/or anticipated outcome that is applied to relatively complex or unstructured ideas for which there is not an obvious solution. (Moon, 1999, p. 23)

a window through which the practitioner can view and focus self within the context of their own lived experience in ways that enable them to confront, understand and work towards resolving the contradictions within their practice between what is desirable and actual practice. Through the conflict of contradiction, the commitment to realise desirable work and understanding why things are as they are, the practitioner is empowered to take more appropriate action in future situations. (Johns, 2000, p. 34)

The above constitute only a few of the definitions available and you are encouraged to further your reading to make an informed choice of your preferred stance. This will depend on your philosophical standpoint and how you view 'knowledge' and 'truth'. You may take the viewpoint that reality is all around us, the sky is blue and the grass is green, we can hear and read about realities and knowledge is acquired by this. However, many would argue that this relies on our 'senses', with authors suggesting that alterations of these senses can distort our view of the world; what we 'expect' to be normal is turned upside down (Newberg and Waldman, 2006; Jahn and Dunne, 2004). Therefore, many theorists suggest that we are ruled by what we 'expect' to see, with our perceptions guided by these expectations. Many philosophers including Kant, Hume, Popper and Fichte have debated the concepts of knowledge, truth and reality with conflicting conclusions, suggesting that these can only be concluded by each individual (Popper, 1979; Fichte, 1982; Guyer and Wood, 1998; Hume, 2008).

An alternative view is that there is no reality, we construct truth individually within our own thinking and this may change with time as our perceptions of society and the world change.

> *The question we should ask ourselves is not 'is this true' but rather 'who decides whether this is true'*. (Rolfe et al., 2001, p. 4)

Depending on your standpoint, reflection will take on a different meaning and how you approach this may differ from colleagues. It is not within this chapter's remit to debate the philosophical and epistemological aspects of truth and knowledge although it would be beneficial to take some time to read around these areas as indicated within the suggested reading list at the end of this chapter, in order to inform your thinking.

You may have already come across varying methods and literature relating to reflection and reflective practice, some of which may seem confusing. New conceptualizations of reflection which acknowledge and value a range of perspectives, contexts and dimensions can be drawn upon to inform your reflective practice (Cotton, 2001). Reflective practice should not be seen as just complying and conforming to organisational and educational requirements, or a method of surveillance. Essentially, you need to focus on *why* you are reflecting in your professional role and what the benefits will be for you, your clients/patients and carers, your organisation and the wider healthcare arena.

You may have been asked to reflect on study days you have attended or workshops where learning has occurred to improve an area of practice. Whilst this might be termed 'reflection', it may only require you to evaluate the session in relation to the meeting of learning outcomes for the session, if you felt the session met your learning needs, and what you will now do with this increased learning – i.e. action plan for practice. An academic assignment that requires critical reflection may expect you to write a fuller analysis of issues relating to the area of study, relating to current and relevant literature in order to structure your thoughts accordingly.

Essentially, there are two methods advocated for critical reflection as described by Schön (1983): *reflection in action* and *reflection on action*. He suggests that reflection on action is for the more novice or intermediate practitioner and reflection in action is associated more with advanced practice due to the more complex roles involved, wealth of experience and in-depth knowledge base, which encourages a critical theorising of issues whilst actually doing them. In reality, it is only you as the practitioner who can justify why and when you reflect and many will feel they already reflect in action within their everyday practice, even though they may be relatively inexperienced. Benner et al. (1999) discuss a similar concept of 'thinking in action' although this is described as narrative understanding from previous patterns of behaviour rather than critical reflection, and therefore does not particularly support any theorising in rationalising judgments within a situation.

It is important to remember that the difference between our personal *thoughts* we have concerning events and *critical reflection* is that critical reflection is a formal process which is explicit and develops knowledge and understanding, distinguishing it from a process of casual thinking. It allows you to analyse why you and others behave the way they do, and situations could be improved if behaviours were changed in future situations (Fook and Gardner, 2007). Reflection can therefore be utilised to continually improve understanding and performance, rather than merely to justify actions that have been taken.

Aims of reflection

- To recognise what we already know
- To identify what we need to learn to increase understanding and knowledge
- To make sense of new understanding and knowledge in the context of the specific experience
- To guide future learning and development

In its simplest form, reflection can be seen as essential to the learning cycle as in Figure 5.1.

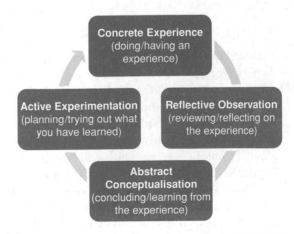

Figure 5.1   Kolb's experiential learning cycle. Adapted from Kolb (1984).

Reflection on action

Reflection on action is concerned with generating and articulating practice-based knowledge and usually occurs after a situation or incident, away from that particular setting.

This type of reflection is about looking at details of a situation or incident in detail, critically analysing these by relating to relevant theory to make sense of the situation and have a deeper knowledge and understanding of themselves, the actions taken and decisions made. This may also include looking at the broader picture, considering influences that may have had an impact on the incident such as communication, organisational approaches/restrictions, teamwork/collaborative working and even political drivers. From this analysis, you will have generated further knowledge in order to improve practice and be able to formulate action plans to address similar situations you may encounter in the future.

Remember reflection is not always about revisiting situations where things have not gone the way you planned, or an incident that has caused you concern. It also relates to sharing 'good' practice, where you can reflect on situations where the care and management of an incident or care episode can be analysed to evaluate why it worked so well, in order to confirm areas of good practice. This then can be disseminated to others in the team/organisation etc. to promote practice improvement.

Varying models of reflection have been advocated to help in the structure of writing a critical reflection and will be discussed later in this chapter. This type of reflection is also useful for mentors to help look at details for professional development with their learners, encouraging them to consider different ways of looking at the problem, develop actions plans and monitor progression.

Reflection in action

In contrast to *reflection on action* which is concerned with post-event analysis, *reflection in action* is concerned with reflection whilst 'doing' (Schön, 1983). This is advocated for advanced practitioners who can utilise this approach to improve their professional practice significantly. Many practitioners would argue that they adopt this approach unconsciously, without necessarily thinking that it is reflection, but considering it as part of their professional advancement and expertise. However, this is not just about technical expertise and skill sets gained throughout their career. Reflection in action combines thinking and doing simultaneously. You may have experienced situations where you can stop and describe that situation, knowing why the situation is as it is, and what needs to be done and why. This is different to how Benner (1984) may describe 'intuition' of

Table 5.1   Advantages and disadvantages of reflection

Advantages	Potential disadvantages
Personal and professional development	Used primarily to look backwards
Learning from mistakes	Can be focused on negative situations
Continuous improvement	Ethical and moral dilemmas can be raised
Improve patient/client care	
Employer/organisation awareness	Uncomfortable feelings/anxiety
Promote the profession	Issues of confidentiality
Sharing good practice	A requirement rather than choice

professionals without conscious thought. Reflection in action is the process of *knowing in action*, with the practitioner

> *being aware of the thoughts and reflections that underpin their clinical judgments and decisions and also of the ways by which they arrive at those thoughts and reflections.* (Rolfe et al., 2001, p. 135)

Discussion point

From your understanding and previous experiences so far, take a few minutes to think about how you now feel about reflection. Write some of the advantages and disadvantages of reflective practice that you consider important when engaging in a reflective process. Table 5.1 gives some examples to get you thinking. Explore and discuss the lists you have compiled with your mentor and/or colleagues; do they agree? what are their views?

Group reflection

Discussing reflection as a group can be beneficial in gaining confidence with the reflective process, so you might want to arrange a 'reflection group' with your peers or fellow students. You may be surprised to learn that members of the group have the same concerns or difficulties with the reflective process such as which model to use, how to ensure the academic levelness of the reflection etc. and you can also gain inspiration from those in the group who may have already mastered the process (Norman, 2008).

Johns (2009) suggests that reflection can be difficult to grasp initially without expert help and support. Encouraging your colleagues to participate in a group reflection can be an opportunity to talk through issues and check your own perceptions within a supportive, non-judgemental, constructive environment. Obviously, ground rules for the group must be formulated in order that confidentiality is maintained with all members agreeing to be honest and open, and appropriate challenging of practice being encouraged to promote development and improvement. Remember alternative viewpoints can provide a valuable learning experience, but there should be no 'right' or 'wrong'. Other ways that groups can reflect can be through action learning sets, PBL and clinical supervision.

Action learning

Action learning sets are essentially workplace groups that meet regularly to discuss problems and collectively explore solutions in order to decide on the best action to take. However, they are becoming increasingly popular in the form of learning sets within academia with many programmes of study incorporating this method of learning into the curriculum. Stages of action learning sets include the following:

- Describing the problem as we see it
- Receiving contributions from others in the form of questions
- Reflecting on our discussion and deciding what action to take
- Reporting back on what happened when we took action
- Reflecting on the problem-solving process and how well it is working

Action learning sets should be facilitated in a small group to ensure everyone has an opportunity to be involved and engage with the process, between 5 and 10 is suggested (Pedler, 2008). Participants are learning all the time, whatever their role in the set: presenter, questioner, active listener or reflector. Action learning can also be a benefit to the organisation by promoting an active learning culture of questioning and seeking new ways of working (McGill and Beaty, 2001).

Guidelines for forming an action learning set

- Agree ground rules about how you will work together
- Share the time planned so that everyone gets a turn
- Each member presents, i.e. briefly describes a problem/situation they would like to discuss
- The group helps the person to explore the problem by reflecting on presenting issues

- Open questions to be used to challenge the current way of working
- Avoid giving advice
- Ensure an action plan is formulated
- Spend time discussing what has been learned

Problem based learning

PBL has been, and continues to be, successfully implemented in numerous disciplines of higher education such as architecture (Wilkie and Burns, 2003) and law. The history of PBL, however, lies predominantly in the health professions (Barrow and Tamblyn, 1980; Chikotas, 2008) as the common factors among these disciplines are the need to actively apply knowledge to the assessment and care of patients and to identify areas in which further learning would enhance or improve patient care.

A key component of PBL is that it is firmly grounded in reality by presenting the group with scenarios that is cognisance of the real world practice. This encourages a deeper learning which is relevant to practice that would foster a multidisciplinary approach, rather than focussing exclusively on a clinical perspective. Another key element of PBL is that it encourages individual or groups to think about clinical practice and how to approach challenging situations, rather than providing the answers.

The goal of PBL is the learning in comparison to problem solving where the outcome is important; the problem provides the context within which learning takes place (Gibbs, 1992). The process is about gaining new knowledge through the process of acquiring information, handling information and giving information (Eraut, 1994). These processes are similar to self-directed learning behaviours (Blumberg and Michael, 1991), which are essential for lifelong learning skills and critical thinking skills for reflective practice.

As with action learning, the group should set ground rules of how the group will work and the problem is then given. Following this, Chiou-Fen et al. (2010) identify five stages in the PBL process which are similar to the stages for action learning. These are as follows:

- Analysis of problems
- Establishment of learning objectives
- Collection of information
- Summarising
- Reflection

The group return to share the agreed learning objectives. The process continues until the group has exhausted all learning opportunities relating to the case study.

Clinical supervision

Over the decade, clinical supervision was introduced into the UK nursing practice as an idea to be developed. Since the introduction, it is now widely used in other health professionals such as midwifery (Kirkham, 1996; Thomas, 2005), mental health professions (Ask and Roche, 2005) and those allied to nursing such as social work (Brown and Bourne, 1996) and occupational therapy (Sweeney et al., 2001).

As a useful concept in these professions, there has been an introduction of several frameworks in existence that guide the process of clinical supervision. The frameworks should help to clarify the process of this to give some direction of what is to be done and to have a sense of what we are aiming at, so that we know where we should be going. Without such clarity, supervision is less likely to be helpful or effective (Van Ooijen, 2003). It is beyond the scope of this chapter to explore these frameworks in detail; however, in its simplest, clinical supervision is a regular and formalised reflective practice between two healthcare professionals.

Driscoll (2007) suggests that reflection is not all of the clinical supervision, but the act of clinical supervision potentiates reflective practice. Through the process of reflection that takes place in clinical supervision, it encourages the healthcare practitioner to look at their practice in a different way that would encourage both healthcare professionals to maintain and improve practice (Van Ooijen, 2003). This process would be equally useful to involve interactions between the individual practitioner and other members of the healthcare team as 'each of us sees the work through the window of his thoughts' (Chakravarti, 1997, p. 1); therefore, it is very useful to acknowledge the views of others.

Driscoll (2007) identified three main components of supervision which is summarised as:

1. *Supervised practice and learning* – this focuses on the skills and attributes required by an individual to become a newly qualified and accountable practitioner
2. *Organisational supervision* – once that individual becomes qualified, this is largely concerned with the maintenance of a professional level of performance which is defined by thought of the policies and standards, job descriptions and the joint setting of performance objectives and appraisals.
3. *Supportive supervision* – informal, ad hoc conversations that emerge spontaneously between colleagues that you can trust. Butterworth (1998) describes an example of informal peer support – the 'tea break/tear break'. This is used as a way of letting colleagues share in the stressful clinical experiences which affects their working day and play a vital part in coping with everyday clinical practice.

> **Discussion point**
>
> Consider the above components of clinical supervision and your experience of clinical supervision. Which component would you consider to be the most effective? Do you use all three components? If not, which component is more widely used by you? Did you use a framework? If not, would a framework give you some direction to your discussion? Was this approach effective? Did it encourage you to change your viewpoint? If so, then how? Did your practice improve as a direct result of clinical supervision?

Reflective writing and models of reflection

Many health professionals and students initially struggle to write a reflective account. It is more comfortable to think things through in our own minds rather than physically writing our thoughts down, analysing meaning and evaluating in order to move things forward in some way. Many students who are required to produce a reflective assignment ask familiar questions:

How many words should it be?
Do I need to use a reflective model and if so which one should I use?
Can I write in the first person?
How many references do I need to use?

Always check with your module tutor relating to academic assignments as answers to the above will vary between programmes of study. Usually reflective writing will adopt the first person:

I was working within my practice area … I felt this could have been improved … I did not foresee this …

or using a combination of first and third person:

… although I felt uncomfortable with the situation, Platzer et al. (2000) described this as a limitation which also concurs with previous literature suggesting that students need to feel in control.

As this type of reflective account will need to fulfil learning outcomes, these should be closely adhered to when planning your assignment. Confirm which marking/grading criteria will be applied in this instance with regard to academic level, and how this relates to your plan, i.e. you will need to identify the level of analysis and synthesis needed. Many students initially feel more confident in writing the descriptive phase of their reflective writing. Many models of reflection (Gibbs, 1988; Driscoll, 2000; Johns, 2000) have this element within their framework and can be useful in revisiting the situation. Conversely, this descriptive element is not the learning focus, so be careful not to write numerous pages on this, you may waste valuable wordage! A succinct account is required as the important elements needed are your analysis of the incident/situation, including how you felt then and now, considering and relating relevant theory to support your understanding and thinking of the situation, and how your increased knowledge and learning will now be applied to practice. However, as previously discussed, reflection is not just about academia, it is concerned with you realising learning and uncovering knowledge as part of your professional practice and requirements.

As humans, our preferred form of communicating is verbal and forms our practice, and therefore many will prefer to utilise methods of reflection groups as discussed above. Nevertheless, reflective writing can be an enlightening and powerful process where you can write purposefully in order to make sense of a situation and learn from your experiences. Rolfe et al. (2001) describe this as *writing to learn* and can have a significant effect on your practice, developing new insights and perceptions and a deeper more critical understanding of the issues involved.

Models of reflection can help to structure your thoughts when writing, especially if you have had little exposure to critical reflection. These models give stages or steps to follow to highlight areas you should be thinking about to include within your reflection. They can vary from simplistic models with relatively few steps to follow, to more complex types which identify a number of questions or stages that need to be addressed within the reflective writing. When using a reflective model to structure your writing, you may find it beneficial to use subheadings related to the differing stages identified.

It is advisable to use a variety of models or frameworks initially to broaden your learning and understanding of reflection. Subsequently, you may decide that one model particularly suits your writing style or you feel more comfortable with, which is the one that you are more likely to use in future work. However, when you feel more confident, you may wish to '*draw*' on a model but not particularly utilise every prescribed stage, you may even decide not to use a model when you are experienced in the critical reflective process, as this may seem too restrictive for certain types of reflective writing such as case studies. It is important to note of the reflective writing is part of an academic assignment, if you state you are utilising a named model or framework, you need to adhere to all stages involved as you may be penalised if you omit these. Otherwise, you could clearly state within the introduction that you will only be *drawing* on this model to structure your analysis and give the reasons why, including a rationale for the choice of model.

Many reflective writers initially make the mistake of *describing* the event in too much detail, as this can seem the easiest stage of the model and one that you feel more comfortable with. However, as discussed earlier, the essence of reflective writing is concerned with learning from the experience and critically analysing the associated issues in order to improve practice. Consequently, it is the *analysis* component of reflective writing that is of more importance. From this, synthesis of ideas can occur and action points for future practice can be developed. There are a range of reflective models and frameworks that you could consider using. Reflective models/frameworks of Gibbs (1998), Driscoll (2000) and Johns (2000) are commonly used, although there are many other models available which you may want use.

Gibbs' reflective model

Gibbs' (1988) cycle of reflection (Figure 5.2) is similar to Kolb's learning cycle (Figure 5.1), as it is a continuous process which can be revisited at various points of your learning journey. It has structured questions which will help you process your reflective thoughts and you may want to use it initially to 'thought shower' ideas and words that are in the forefront of your mind immediately following an incident or situation. You can then revisit these initial thoughts and use the cycle to further critically reflect

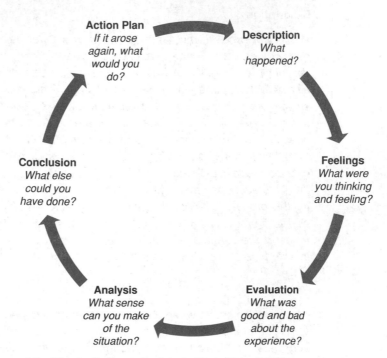

Action Plan
If it arose again, what would you do?

Description
What happened?

Conclusion
What else could you have done?

Feelings
What were you thinking and feeling?

Analysis
What sense can you make of the situation?

Evaluation
What was good and bad about the experience?

Figure 5.2   Gibbs' reflective cycle. Adapted from Gibbs (1988).

on the wider issues involved. The model was initially used within education but has been adopted by many professions as the model of choice for simple, structured reflective practice. However, in order to retain criticality, care must be taken when writing to ensure this is not too descriptive. You can do this by ensuring analysis is evident throughout the stages, not just within the 'analysis' section indicated.

The following is an example of reflective writing from clinical practice that utilises Gibbs' 1988 model of reflection:

Reflective Writing

I am currently a paramedic student and the following reflective writing is based on my experience of attempting to insert a peripheral intravenous (IV) cannulation whilst on my practice placement in the pre-hospital setting. My aims of this refection are to focus on my reasons for failing to insert an IV cannula only. I will use Gibbs (1988) model as this allows me to explore my feelings and analyse the situation and also to enable me to keep focused solely on my objective. As a paramedic student, I am supervised at all times by a registered paramedic or paramedic mentor. To maintain confidentiality of my colleagues and patients, no names will be used (Data Protection Act 1998; Health and Care Professions Council (HCPC), 2012).

Description

Whilst working with my paramedic mentor we were alerted via Emergency Operations Centre to attend a 78-year-old male who was having difficulty breathing. We arrived on scene and the patient had been in bed all day feeling "generally unwell and chesty". A primary and secondary survey which included a full medical history was conducted. Following a clinical examination, my mentor informed me that the patient would need to have an IV cannula inserted as a prophylactic measure and that I was to insert this into the patient. The whole process of inserting an IV cannula was explained to the patient. The patient was also informed that I was a student paramedic and that my mentor would supervise me during this process. The patient gave his verbal consent for me to continue with this procedure. On two attempts of this procedure I was unable to insert the cannula and my mentor then took over and successfully inserted the cannula into the patient on his first attempt.

Feelings

I was really pleased when my mentor asked me to perform this skill as I had not attempted this skill in practice yet. I was very excited yet also very nervous. I had the theory taught in the university and practiced using mannequines. Initially I felt it was difficult at practising on the mannequines. This was due to the handling of the cannula and the technique of inserting it into a vein at the same time as holding the patient's upper limb. With practice this did get easier and I felt confident in my ability to practice this safely. I was also assured by the lecturers that it was more difficult on a manikin due to the thickness of the plastic skin and difficulty holding the equipment. However, the lecturers also said that it can be more difficult performing this skill on patients due to various reasons such as the patient moving their limb when inserting cannula, patients fainting, veins collapsing are just a few to mention.

I felt nervous because it was my first time doing this skills in a real situation, and it had been 3 weeks ago when this was taught in university. I wondered if I would be able to remember everything such as gaining consent, infection control, health and safety, which cannula and vein to use and handling the equipment. I also felt slightly intimidated by my mentor watching over me. I had worked with my mentor previously and we had developed a good working relationship which is essential for effective student learning (Nursing and Midwifery Council (NMC), 2008) so I couldn't understand why I felt this way. Yet, despite this I also felt reassured knowing that my mentor was there, to discuss the procedure and support and guide me through this challenging situation which is key characteristic of the mentor role (Darling, 1984). Despite the support and guidance, unfortunately I failed to insert the IV cannula on two occasions and this made me feel totally distraught. This was my first attempt at this skill and failing on two attempts made a significant impact on my confidence as I felt completely inadequate of not being able to do this, especially as my mentor successfully inserted the cannula on his first attempt.

Evaluation

What was good about the experience was that I communicated to the patient to fully explain the reasons for inserting the IV cannula and that I was a student paramedic being supervised by my mentor. This was important as I needed to obtain informed consent to continue with this procedure. This is a legal and professional requirement of a paramedic before any treatment is carried out as the Health and Care Professions Council (HCPC) (2012, p. 12) state that as a registrant "you must explain to the service user the treatment you are planning to provide". This is to ensure the patient is fully informed to get their informed consent (HCPC, 2012). The patient was fully aware of the procedure due his previous experiences as a service user and consent was given.

On attempting this skill, unfortunately I failed this on two occasions and apart from being very nervous I could not think of any reasons why I failed. Prior to this, I felt confident with most aspects of clinical care in the pre-hospital environment and felt I was developing my knowledge and skills. However, this experience was not a positive learning experience for me as I felt totally inadequate and incompetent. I was very upset and disappointed with myself; however, following constructive feedback with my mentor I reflected upon the incident and explored the reasons why I was not able to cannulate the patient.

Analysis

In the pre-hospital environment, there two methods of gaining vascular access; peripheral intravenous (IV) access and intraosseous (IO) access. IV access using a cannula (venflon) inserted into a peripheral vein of the upper limb is generally the route of choice (Gregory and Ward, 2010). IV cannulation is indicated for administration of fluids, administration of drugs and to obtain blood specimens for testing in a laboratory. Another indication for IV access is for prophylactic measures and due to the acuteness of the patient's clinical condition; the patient was cannulated for this purpose.

There are potential complications associated with IV cannulation, and insertion of an IV cannula for prophylactic reasons should be discouraged (Gregory and Murcell, 2010). However, in certain circumstances, this should be considered (Gregory and Ward, 2010). The patient could have deteriorated very rapidly and therefore the decision to cannulate the patient was clearly justified. The HCPC (2012) state that paramedics must recognise that they are personally responsible. As an accountable practitioner 'you must be able to justify your decisions if asked to' (HCPC, 2012, p. 8).

It is important to identify the indications for IV access so that the smallest size is used for the intended purpose (Cox and Roper, 2009). IV cannulas have a colour-coded port with a cap which corresponds to the size. The sizes range from 22 gauge being the smallest to 14 gauge being the largest. Using 14 gauge or 16 gauge should be used in urgent situations where large volumes of colloid or blood are required very quickly, 18 gauge for blood components or large amount of fluid and 22 gauge and 20 gauge should be used for neonates, fragile vein and longer term medication (Cox and Roper, 2009). Generally, 18 gauge and 20 gauge are used in the pre-hospital setting as they will fulfil most functions.

It is also important to identify the choice of vein to ensure the correct size of cannula is selected. The size of the device should fit in the vein and allow a good blood flow around the outside of the vein to reduce the risk of mechanical phlebitis. This is caused by the size of the external diameter of the cannula being greater than the vessel lumen which irritates the vessel walls (Dougherty and Lister, 2008). Due to their superior blood flow, the veins in the upper limb are more suitable for cannulation than the lower limb. Peripheral veins of the upper limb with the larger veins located into the anterior region of the elbow (also known as anticubital fossa region) and the smaller veins in the dorsal aspect of the hand. The forearm is considered a suitable vein for cannulation but this area is frequently overlooked, and as splinting is unnecessary in this area, it is quite comfortable for the patient (Royal College of Nursing (RCN) (2006)). The non-dominant limb should be used and when possible avoidance of insertion over a joint. This will reduce the risk of mechanical phlebitis and disruption of flow of fluids and drugs which is caused by movement. Veins over bony prominence should also be avoided to reduce pain and discomfort. Other factors to consider when choosing a suitable vein are limb injuries, other clinical procedures to the limb, infection, arteriovenous fistulae, stroke, lymphadenopathy, current IV drug therapy, age of the patient, patient cooperation/previous experience, previous uses of vein and the patient's weight, i.e. obese or malnourished. Gregory and Murcell (2010) suggest that the initial attempt should be made at the distal end of the limb as unsuccessful attempts hinder the use of veins distal to the original site. On examination of the patient's hand, his skin was very fragile and his veins were very tortuous and mobile due to his age. When selecting a vein it should be soft, bouncy, visible and palpable, and refill when depressed and well supported by subcutaneous tissue (Dougherty, 2006). A 20-gauge cannula was selected to insert into his cephalic vein of his forearm.

On insertion of the cannula I was very nervous and as I inserted this I was not able to get a flashback of blood on both occasions. It was at that point my mentor took over and proceeded to successfully insert the cannula. Gregory and Murcell (2010) suggest that no more than 2 attempts should be made and wherever possible cannulation should be done en route to hospital to prevent delay in treatment. As previously stated, I was extremely disappointed at failing this skill which at that time made me feel inadequate and I lost my confidence. I didn't fully understand why I failed but I could only blame myself and lack of experience for causing this. Elliot (2010) suggests that local complications can occur during cannulation which include, infiltration, vasoconstriction and haematoma formation. As the patient did not have a haematoma, vasoconstriction or infiltration could have been the probable causes.

Infiltration is a mechanical failure as a result of the cannula being inserted too far by the operator causing the needle to puncture through the outer walls of the vein (Elliot, 2010). Caroline (2007) states that many paramedics develop their own individual techniques; however, if it is a continuous problem, inserting a cannula without the aid of a venous tourniquet is suggested (Caroline, 2007). It can also be caused by fluid leakage into the tissues but as there was no fluids administered this was ruled out. Vasoconstriction can also be caused by mechanical failure due to poor technique. This is caused by stimulus (from the cannula) to the tunica media or the valve which causes the smooth muscle to contract and subsequently collapsing the vein. Patient anxiety, temperature, hypovolaemia, dehydration or chemical irritation can also be contributory to vasoconstriction (RCN, 2006). The patient did not feel hot or cold and was not hypovolaemic or dehydrated and therefore this was ruled as a cause of failed attempts. I did consider patient anxiety as this can cause the patient to be tense which affects the smooth muscle of tunica media. However, this was quickly ruled out as I had fully explained this procedure to the patient to reduce his anxiety and the patient had previous experience of being cannulated. After deducting possible causes, I concluded that vasoconstriction caused by mechanical irritation through poor technique was the reason I wasn't able to insert the IV device.

Conclusion

From analysing the situation, it was apparent that my nervousness throughout this experience was a result of my poor technique. As a student paramedic, my knowledge of practicing this skill was on a mannequin and although I felt confident following this, I didn't expect to feel as nervous inserting this into a patient's vein. At the time of the incident there was nothing else I could have done to resolve this situation, however, I can use this negative experience and turn it around to a positive learning experience. The positive aspects are that it was a valuable experience and a learning curve as it encouraged me to not only review the literature around intravenous cannulation; but I have also explored the literature around strategies that I can apply to situation to enable me to cope with stressful situations to reduce my anxiety and nervousness. This will prepare me for future situations both as a paramedic student and when I qualify as a registered paramedic.

Action Plan

This is a short-term plan for the duration of my 12-week placement:

- *Review the literature wider to ensure I have a deep knowledge and understanding of intravenous cannulation*
- *Discuss any concerns I have with my mentor*
- *Practice my technique in the training school with my mentor*
- *Apply strategies to reduce anxiety*
- *To continue to take all opportunities to practice the skill under supervision of my mentor to achieve a competent level by the end of my placement.*

Johns' reflective model

Johns' (2000) reflective model identifies 'ways of knowing'; aesthetics, *personal*, *ethics*, *empirics* and *reflexivity*, which are based on Carper's (1978) four patterns of knowing (for further discussion, see Chapter 3). This model of reflection is a more complex framework which requires further detail in order to address the reflective cues proposed.

Aesthetics

Reflective cues

- Bring the mind home
- Focus on a description of an experience that seems significant in some way
- What particular issues seem significant to pay attention to?
- How others are feeling and what made me were feel that way?
- What was I trying to achieve and did I respond effectively?
- What were the consequences of my actions on the patient, others and me?

Personal

- How was I feeling and what made me feel that way?

Ethics

- To what extent did I act for the best and in tune with my values?

Empirics

- What knowledge did or might have informed me?

Reflexivity

- How does this situation connect with previous experiences?
- How might I respond more effectively given this situation again?
- What would be the consequences of alternative actions for the patient, others and myself?
- How do I now feel about this experience?
- Am I more able to support myself and others better as a consequence?
- Am I more able to realise desirable practice monitored using appropriate frameworks such as framing perspectives, Carper's fundamental ways of knowing and other maps?

Johns (2000)

Johns (2000) suggests using the framework as a guide to structure a learning diary, although this may not be particular requirement for your reflection. If using this model within an academic assignment, using subheadings for the numerous reflective cues proposed may detract from the flow of your writing.

Discussion point

The example of reflective writing used for Gibbs' (1988) reflective model was very limited as this focused on the causes of a failed attempt when inserting an IV cannula. Imagine this scenario and you are asked to write a reflective patient case study. Using the reflect clues in Johns' (2000) model of reflection other than describing your experience, feelings, what other issues could you reflect upon? Does this model provide more structure and cues to explore this in more detail?

Consider the following issues that can arise in a reflective patient case study. How would you relate this to the reflective clues?

- Primary and Secondary Survey
- History Taking
- Communication
- Pathophysiology of the patient's condition
- IV drug therapy for the patient's clinical condition
- Was there an alternative to IV drug therapy?
- Consent
- How did the patient feel? What are the consequences of your actions on the patient and others?
- Professional accountability and your values
- The role of the mentor? How did your mentor feel?

Driscoll's reflective model

Driscoll's (2000) model of reflection has its origins in clinical supervision, with the model encouraging a structured reflective approach to the clinical supervision encounter, suggesting that reflective practice is essential for this process. Driscoll (2000) suggests that the process of reflection and clinical supervision is inextricably linked. The three main questions identified to structure your reflective writing are *What? So What?* and *Now What?* and include additional trigger questions as illustrated below to encourage further exploration. Driscoll (2007, p. 27) states that 'the questions are intended to emphasise practitioner learning and the subsequent actions that arise from them'.

What? Returning to the situation

What is the purpose of returning to this situation?
What exactly occurred?
What did you see and what did you do?
What was your reaction?
What did other people do? e.g. colleagues/patient
What do you see as key aspects of this situation?

So what? Understanding the context

What were you feeling at the time?
What are you feeling now? Are there any differences and if so why?
What were the effects of what you did (or did not do)?
What good emerged from the situation? e.g. for self and others
What troubles you if anything?
What were your experiences in comparison to your colleagues?
What are the reasons for feeling differently from your colleagues?

Now what? Modifying future outcomes

What are the implications for you?
What needs to happen to alter the situation?
What are you going to do about the situation?
What happens if you decide not to alter anything?
What might you do differently next time?
What information do you need to face a similar situation again?
What are the best ways of getting information about the situation should it arise again?

> **Critical thinking**
>
> Now consider a positive experience from clinical practice that you have shared with your peers or mentor. Consider why you choose that incident to reflect upon (What?) and link this to the reflective cues in Driscoll's model. Did your discussion follow this structure? If not, discuss the same incident with your peers using this model. Did this encourage a deeper reflective discussion?

Summary

Reflection and reflective practice is now a fundamental part of health-care practice and all healthcare professionals are required to use reflective practice as part of their professional requirements. This chapter has introduced the key concepts of reflection and reflective practice to enable you to increase your understanding of reflection, the benefits of reflection and how you can apply this to practice. You will all be at different points in your professional career but the benefits of reflection will apply to each point of your professional journey as the benefits of reflection will increase new knowledge, increase your theoretical understanding which will bridge the theory practice gap, identify ways to improve your practice and develop your professional skills and attitude.

When embarking on the reflective process, there are a variety of methods that will support this. You may choose to have an informal or formal one-to-one discussion or group discussion and the methods in this chapter have demonstrated which method will be most appropriate to use. Reflective writing is considered the most challenging method, yet, there are a range of reflective models that will guide and structure your reflective writing. Some models you will find very easy to follow, but other models can be very complex which are demonstrated in this chapter. It is important to choose the appropriate model for the purpose of your reflection as 'not one size fits all'.

When writing a reflective piece of work, it is very easy to get caught up in describing the event rather than critically analysing, and subsequently, the essence of the reflective process is lost. The example of reflective writing and discussion points will show you that by using different reflective models, will enable you to be more self-aware and encourage you to solve the problem and start thinking more critically, which will promote a deeper learning experience.

References

Ask, A. & Roche, A. (2005) *Clinical Supervision: A Practical Guide for the Alcohol and Other Drugs Field*. National Centre for Education and Training on Addiction (NCETA) and Flinder University, Adelaide.

Atkins, S. & Murphy, K. (1994) Reflective practice. *Nursing Standard*, **8**(39), 49–54.

Barrow, H.S. & Tamblyn, R.M. (1980) *Problem Based Learning: An Approach to Medical Education*. Springer, New York.

Benner, P. (1984) *From Novice to Expert: Excellence and Power in Clinical Nursing Practice*. Addison-Wesley, Boston, MA.

Benner, P., Hooper-Kyriakidis, P. & Stannard, D. (1999) *Clinical Wisdom and Interventions in Critical Care: A Thinking-in-Action Approach*. W.B. Saunders, Philadelphia.

Blumberg, P. & Michael, J. (1991) In: *Developing Learning in Professional Education. Partnerships for Practice* (ed. I. Taylor), p. 95. The Society for Research into Higher Education and Open University Press, Buckingham.

Boyd, E. & Fayles, A. (1983) Reflective learning: key to learning from experience. *Journal of Humanistic Psychology*, **23**, 99–117.

Brown, A. & Bourne, I. (1996) *The Social Work Supervisor*. Open University Press, Milton Keynes.

Butterworth, T. (1998) In: *Clinical Supervision and Mentoring in Nursing*, 2nd edn (eds T. Butterworth, J. Faugier & P. Burnard), pp. 1–18. Stanley Thornes, Cheltenham.

Caroline, N.L. (2007) *Emergency Care in the Streets*, 6th edn. Jones and Bartlett Publishers, London.

Carper, B. (1978) Fundamental patterns of knowing in nursing. *Advances in Nursing Science*, **1**(10), 13–23.

Chakravarti, A. (1997) In: *Clinical Supervision Made Easy* (ed. Els van Ooijen), p. 1. Churchill Livingstone, London.

Chikotas, N.E. (2008) Theoretical links: supporting the use of problem-based learning in the education of the nurse practitioner. *Nursing Education Perspectives*, **29**(6), 359–362.

Chiou-Fen, L., Meei-Shiow, Lu., Chun-Chih, C. & Che-Ming, Yang. (2010) A comparison of problem-based learning and conventional teaching in nursing ethics education. *Nursing Ethics*, **17**(3), 373–382.

Cotton, A. (2001) Private thoughts in public spheres: issues in reflection and reflective practices in nursing. *Journal of Advanced Nursing*, **36**(4), 512–519.

Cox, N.T. & Roper, T.A. (2009) *Clinical Skills*. Oxford University Press, Oxford.

Darling, L.A.W. (1984) 'What do nurses want in a mentor? *Journal of Nursing Administration*, **14**(10), 42–44.

Data Protection Act (1998) *The National Archives*. Available at http://www.legislation.gov.uk (accessed 4 January 2012).

Dewey, J. (1933) *How We Think: A Restatement of the Relation of Reflective Thinking to the Educative Process*. Henry Regnery, Chicago.

Dougherty, L (2006) *Central Venous Access Devices: Care and Management (Essential Clinical Skills for Nurses)*. Blackwell Publishing, Oxford.

Dougherty, L. & Lister, S (2008) *The Royal Marsden Hospital Manual of Clinical Nursing Procedures*. Blackwell Publishing, Oxford.

Driscoll, J. (2000) *Practising Clinical Supervision: A Reflective Approach*. Baillière Tindall, London.

Driscoll, J. (2007) *Practicing Clinical Supervision: A Reflective Approach for Healthcare Professionals*, 2nd edn. Baillière Tindall, London.

Elliot, T.S.J. (2010) *A Guide to Peripheral Intravenous Cannulation*. Ohmeda, Hatfield.

Eraut, M. (1994) *Developing Professional Knowledge and Competence*. Falmer, London.

Fichte, J.G. (1982) *The Science of Knowledge*. Cambridge University Press, Cambridge.

Fook, J. & Gardner, F. (2007) *Practising Critical Reflection: A Resource Handbook*. Open University Press, Berkshire.

Gibbs, G. (1988) *Learning by Doing: A Guide to Teaching and Learning Methods*. Further Education Unit, Oxford Polytechnic, Oxford.

Gibbs, G. (1992) Improving the quality of student learning through course design. In: *Learning to Effect* (ed. R. Barnett), p. 157. Open University Press, Buckingham.

Gilbert, T. (2001) Reflective practice and clinical supervision: meticulous rituals of the confessional. *Journal of Advanced Nursing*, **36**(2), 199–205.

Gregory, P. & Murcell, I. (2010) *Manual of Clinical Paramedic Procedures*. Wiley-Blackwell, Chichester.

Gregory, P. & Ward, A. (eds) (2010) *Sanders' Paramedic Textbook*. Elsevier, London.

Gustafsson, C. & Fagerberg, I. (2004) Reflection: the way to professional development? *Journal of Clinical Nursing*, **13**, 271–280.

Guyer, P. & Wood, A.W. (1998) *The Works of Emmanual Kant: Critique of Pure Reason*. Cambridge University Press, Cambridge.

Habermas, J. (1972) *Knowledge and Human Interests*. Heinemann, London.

Hannigan, B. (2001) A discussion of the strengths and weaknesses of 'reflection' in nursing practice and education. *Journal of Clinical Nursing*, **10**(2), 278–283.

Health and Care Professions Council (HCPC) (2012) *Standards of Conduct, Performance and Ethics*. HCPC, London.

Hume, D. (1748) Republished 2008. *An Enquiry Concerning Human Understanding*. Available at http://www.forgottenbooks.org (accessed 31 May 2011).

Jahn, R.G. & Dunne, B.J. (2004) Sensors, filters and the source of reality. *Journal of Scientific Exploration*, **18**(4), 547–570.

Jarvis, P. (1992) Reflective practice in nursing. *Nurse Education Today*, **12**, 174–181.

Johns, C. (2000) *Becoming a Reflective Practitioner*. Blackwell Publishing, Oxford.

Johns, C. (2009) *Becoming a Reflective Practitioner*, 3rd edn. Wiley-Blackwell Publishing, Chichester.

Kirkham, M. (1996) *Supervision of Midwives*. Midwives Press, London.

Kolb, D.A. (1984) *Experiential Learning: Experience as the Source of Learning and Development*. Prentice Hall, New Jersey.

McGill, I. & Beaty, L. (2001) *Action Learning: A Guide for Professional, Management and Educational Development*, 2nd edn. Routledge, London.

Mezirow, J. (1998) On critical reflection. *Adult Education Quarterly*, **45**, 185–198.

Moon, J. (1999) *Learning Journals. A Handbook for Academics, Students and Professional Development*. Kogan Page, London.

Newberg, A. & Waldman, M.R. (2006) *Why We Believe What We Believe*. Free Press, New York.

Norman, K. (ed.) (2008) *Portfolios in the Nursing Profession: Use in Assessment and Professional Development*. Quay Books, London.

Nursing and Midwifery Council (NMC) (2008) *Standards to Support Learning and Assessment in Practice*. NMC, London.

Pedler, M. (2008) *Action Learning for Managers*, 2nd edn. Gower Publishing, Hampshire.

Platzer, H., Blake, D. & Ashford, D. (2000) Barriers to learning from reflection: a study in the use of group work with post registration nurses. *Journal of Advanced Nursing*, **31**(5), 1001–1008.

Popper, K.R. (1979) *Objective Knowledge: An Evolutionary Approach*. Oxford University Press, Oxford.

Reid, B. (1993) 'But we're doing it already' exploring a response to the concept of reflective practice in order to improve its facilitation. *Nurse Education Today*, **13**(4), 305–309.

Rolfe, G., Freshwater, D. & Jasper, M. (2001) *Critical Reflection for Nursing and the Helping Professions: A User's Guide*. Palgrave MacMillan, Hampshire.

Royal College of Nursing (RCN) (2006) *Peripheral Venous Cannulation in Children and Young People*. Available at http://www.rcn.org.uk (accessed 6 February 2012).

Saylor, C. (1990) Reflection and professional education: art, science and competency. *Nurse Educator*, **15**, 8–11.

Schön, D. (1983) *The Reflective Practitioner: How Professionals Think in Action*. Avery Press, Aldershot.

Schön, D. (1991) *Educating the Reflective Practitioner*. Jossey-Bass, San Francisco.

Sweeney, G., Webley, P. & Treacher, A. (2001) Supervision in occupational therapy part 3: accommodating the supervisor and supervisee. *British Journal of Occupational Therapy*, **64**(1), 426–431.

Teekman, B. (2000) Exploring reflective thinking in nursing practice. *Journal of Advanced Nursing*, **31**, 1125–1135.

Thomas, R. (2005) Practice, legal principle and the supervisor. *Practising Midwife*, **8**(8), 22–25.

Van Ooijen, E. (2003) *Clinical Supervision Made Easy*. Churchill Livingstone, London.

Wilkie, K. & Burns, I. (2003) *Problem-Based Learning. A Handbook for Nurses*. Palgrave Macmillan, Hampshire.

Williams, B. (2001) Developing critical reflection for professional practice through problem based learning. *Journal of Advanced Nursing*, **34**(1), 27–34.

6 Professional and Legal Issues

Karen Latcham

Faculty of Health Sciences, Stafford University, Stafford, UK

Introduction

There is now much more awareness for patients within the healthcare arena who can readily access clinical guidelines to inform them of the care that should be received. Combine this with the increase of litigation, it is no surprise that the vagueness and complexity of the law means that professional and legal issues become confusing for healthcare professionals. Much has been written to offer guidance on such broad areas, but it is of paramount importance that healthcare practitioners have an understanding and are mindful of how the law influences their clinical practice, not only to ensure public trust and provide effective care but also to avoid patient harm and legal action.

This chapter aims to provide an insight into the need for professional regulation, why adherence to professional standards ensure that healthcare professionals deliver effective accountable care and why continuous professional development (CPD) is of utmost importance to ensure practitioners remain fit to practice. The discussions will focus on the regulatory standards set by the Health & Care Professions Council (HCPC, formerly the Health Professions Council) which regulates allied health professionals.

We live in a much richer, more risk adverse society than ever before and are much better informed of our rights. Litigation and claims of negligent practice are on the increase which not only creates a massive drain on the National Health Service (NHS) budget but also ultimately impacts on patient care. Reference to professional guidelines, legal frameworks and case law will be used to raise awareness of how negligence claims can be successful.

Caring for such diverse patients makes obtaining patient consent an area of confusion for healthcare practitioners who have a duty to protect not only a patient's vulnerability but also their human rights. Consent for the competent adult, those who lack capacity and children will be addressed

---

Professional Practice in Paramedic, Emergency and Urgent Care, First Edition. Edited by Val Nixon.
© 2013 John Wiley & Sons, Ltd. Published 2013 by John Wiley & Sons, Ltd.

and the legal statutes to protect those with a mental health illness. It will identify the need for practitioners to be vigilant in protecting patient confidentiality and identify when disclosure of confidential information can be given. Finally, the chapter will conclude with a brief discussion of mental capacity, deprivation of a patient's liberty and provide an overview of ethical theories identifying how these are used to resolve ethical dilemmas faced by practitioners within healthcare.

Registration and professional standards

Professional regulation is necessary to ensure healthcare professionals are accountable not only through general law and their contracts of employment but also through a governing body for their profession. The aim of professional regulation is to have set standards for practitioners, to maintain a register of those fit to practice which in turn, protects the public, communicates best practice, and enables the provision of a quality service.

Professional regulation is not a new concept; doctors have been professionally regulated by the General Medical Council (GMC), nurses and midwives by the Nursing and Midwifery Council (NMC) for many years. However, for many years, healthcare professionals that did not fall into a category of doctor, nurse or midwife did not have statutory regulation. This was addressed following the Health Professions Order in 2001 and subsequently, the Health Professions Council (HCPC), an independent UK-wide statutory body was established in April 2002 to safeguard the well-being of persons accessing the services of a registrant. The register opened in July 2003, and currently regulates 17 allied health professions. The introduction of the Health and Social Care Act 2012 has led to the HPC regulating social workers in England. Consequently, the government requested the HPC to change their name. From August 1st 2012, the new name of Health & Care Professions Council came into effect. The HCPC states that not everyone registered by them works in 'health' or 'care', the new name will better describe the diverse range of professions we regulate (HCPC, 2012b). The HCPC set many regulatory standards that registrants are duty bound to adhere to. The standards of conduct, performance and ethics (HCPC, 2012a) are enforced to fulfil its function in promoting high standards of professional conduct making each registered professional accountable for their actions. The standards of proficiency (HCPC, 2012c) are the minimum standards necessary to protect the public, to ensure the professions regulated work safely and effectively. All practitioners must ensure that they meet the expectations of the community and uphold high ethical behaviour.

The clinical role of a paramedic has undergone significant change over the last 20 years and the introduction of registration brings with it the need to understand and adhere to professional standards. Clinical advice and clinical guidelines are given for paramedics by the Joint Royal College

Ambulance Liaison Committee (JRCALC) (2006). If professional practice is questioned, then the regulatory body may hold a professional to account and ask them to justify their actions. The HCPC will consider complaints from members of the public, employers, professionals and the police to protect the public. If someone raises concern about a registrant's practice, then a fitness to practice panel will consider the individual circumstances against the standards to decide whether further action needs taking which may include receiving a caution, placing conditions on their registration, suspension or in serious cases removal from the register. However, if a practitioner's prime concern is in the best interest of the service user and they can justify any decisions, it is very unlikely that you will not meet the standards (HCPC, 2012a).

As a qualified practitioner, you become an autonomous and account-able professional and need to make professional informed decisions about your practice to ensure your commitment to safeguard and protect patient safety. Hence, you have a duty to report a colleague whose conduct you consider may not make them fit to practise, any acts of misconduct or treat-ment provided to a patient that you deem harmful. However, this duty to report does not always happen due to reluctance and fear of harassment or disciplinary action. Yet, what practitioners fail to realise is that by not reporting, they are in breach of not only their professional code of conduct and regulatory frameworks but also often their contract of employment. The laying in statute of the Public Interest Disclosure Act 1998 provides retribution from an employer and protection from unfavourable treatment when raising a concern or whistle blowing.

A further addition to improving standards for registered healthcare pro-fessionals was the implementation of CPD. It is of paramount importance that CPD is carried out to underpin best practice and deliver a quality ser-vice. The HCPC implemented CPD for all registrants in 2006, which be-came a new concept for many of their regulated professions, causing anx-iety and apprehension. All registered healthcare professionals have a duty to update their practice and evidence newly acquired skills and knowl-edge to remain registered and accountable for the delivery of patient care (HCPC, 2012a). A healthcare professional needs to ensure they are familiar with the CPD standards set by the HCPC (2012e) to ensure they meet the standards of proficiency to enable re-registration. (CPD is discussed further in Chapter 9.)

Accountability

All healthcare professionals are accountable to their patients, colleagues, employers through their contract of employment and to their profession through registration, being liable to be held responsible if any acts or omissions lead to ineffective patient care. Accountability is a fundamental concept that is vital for the protection of individual patient needs. Paramedics are accountable for their actions at all times and to their patient and the ambulance service. They encounter vulnerable patients and relatives during critical times and in extremely distressing emergency medical situations where urgent decisions have to be made and immediate action taken. A hurried incorrect decision made in these stressful situations could lead to their accountability being questioned. However, providing the decision and treatment provided is carried out in the patient's best interests in accordance with current legislation, then accountable professional practice should be delivered.

Duty of care

A hospital and its entire staff owe a duty of care to patients admitted for treatment. Following an emergency call, the ambulance service has a duty to respond and provide care. Accident & Emergency (A&E) departments have a duty of care to treat anyone who present themselves and are liable for negligence if they send them away untreated. Hospitals without an A&E facility will display signs stating the location of the nearest A&E department. This ensures that the hospital could not be held negligent if a patient presented and required emergency treatment as the hospital or its staff had never assumed a duty of care. Once a patient is handed over, a duty of care is created between the patient and the practitioner and this cannot be terminated unless the patient no longer requires the care or the carer is replaced by another equally qualified, competent person. It is therefore extremely important that practitioners are aware of their local policies, professional standards and their scope of practice to avoid becoming liable for litigation by putting a patient at risk, delivering ineffective care or breaching their duty of care. The HCPC (2012a, p. 11) informs

> *A registrant must act within the limits of their knowledge, skills and experience and when accepting a service user, have a duty of care. This includes the duty to refer them for further treatment if it becomes clear that the task is beyond a practitioner's scope of practice.*

Clinical negligence

Healthcare relies on a range of complex interactions of people, clinical skills and technology to deliver effective patient care but unfortunately sometimes things go wrong. Complaints have increased with medical mishaps appearing in the press at regular intervals and Brazier and Cave (2007) suggest that we are living in a 'compensation culture'. McHale and Fox (2007) imply that this leads us to question whether doctors are practicing 'defensive medicine' altering their clinical practice to what may be perceived to be safe even though this may not be the most appropriate for the patient based on the basis that the treatment will reduce the risk of the actions.

Patient empowerment is now the order of the day and suing the NHS has become one of the United Kingdom's growth industries. A profitable industry has developed from claiming damages which is evidenced through media commercial advertisements conveying 'No win No fee' slogans. However, those making unsubstantiated claims fail to realise that they ultimately pay the price from increase in taxes plus a financial drain on NHS resources. Conversely, the rise in negligence claims could be considered as having a positive effect towards patient care because organisations fearing the prospect of litigation become duty bound to improve their management of risks and delivery of services.

The NHS through the clinical governance agenda has a duty to provide quality healthcare. One of the strands of clinical governance is clinical risk management which makes providers responsible for the provision of effective healthcare. The flaw with this is that it can impose a greater burden on organisations and the healthcare professional often making us overcautious with decision making. Over recent years, the increase and cost of negligence has dramatically increased the NHS expenditure and this is evidenced by the National Health Service Litigation Authority (NHSLA) (2011) statistics for 2010–2012 (see Table 6.1). To tackle the problem of the rise in negligence claims and the financial demand on NHS resources, the government laid in statute the NHS Redress Act 2006. One of the aims being to provide quick access to redress in relation to liability for services provided as part of health service advocating that an explanation and apology should become part of the clinical process. The scheme is managed by the NHSLA introduced in 1995; one of its key functions is to reduce the number of preventable accidents through an extensive risk management programme. The NHSLA has produced risk management standards for the ambulance service (NHSLA, 2012) and will carry out objective assessments

Table 6.1   NHS clinical negligence claims 2008–2011

Year	Clinical negligence claims	Non-clinical negligence claims	Cost (million)
2008–2009	6080	3743	£769
2009–2010	6652	4074	£787
2010–2011	8655	4346	£863

Data from National Health Service Litigation Authority (NHSLA) (2011) *The National Health Service Litigation Authority. Reports and Accounts 2010–11.*
http://www.nhsla.com/AboutUs/Documents/NHSLA Annual Report and Accounts 2011.pdf

to establish compliance with the set standards. They will review organisation documentation, health records, staff training records, evidence in practice and interview staff to assess their knowledge of the documents and processes (NHSLA, 2012).

To avoid a health authority meeting the costs from litigation, the Clinical Negligence Scheme for Trusts (CNST) was set up in 1995 which is managed by the NHSLA. The premiums for NHS trusts are calculated on the services and scale of operations they perform. To enable an NHS trust to become part of the CNST, they must comply and adhere to the risk management set by CNST.

What is clinical negligence?

The Civil law of negligence provides compensation to a patient if injured by neglect. It is not only physical harm but litigation can also arise from psychiatric harm. Criminal negligence may be punished by criminal courts and occurs when a professional becomes indifferent to the safety of a patient or the value of their life. Mason and McCall Smith (2011) inform that this is effectively limited to prosecutions of manslaughter. It is therefore paramount that healthcare professionals are aware of their scope of practice, regulatory frameworks and their code of conduct that informs a healthcare professional to only take on an intervention that they are competent to perform. The HCPC (2012a) inform that when accepting a service user, you have a duty of care and if the care needed is outside their capabilities and scope of practice, then a duty to refer for further treatment arises.

Proving clinical negligence is based on three key elements (see Box 6.1) and the law and negligence require that all three elements must be established before a claim for compensation will succeed. As previously identified, a duty of care arises when a patient is handed over to a healthcare professional, if an untoward incident or harm has occurred which has led to a litigation claim, the first two elements are easy to prove. It is the third element, the causation of the incident, that also has to be satisfied. If we look at the case in Box 6.2, it will reinforce how causation is central to a successful claim.

Box 6.1   Standards for establishing negligence in UK law

1. A duty of care was owed.
2. The duty and standard of care was breached.
3. The claimant has to prove that the standard of care given failed to reach the acceptable standard given by their peers (Causation).

Bolam v. Friern Hospital Management Committee [1957] 2 All ER 118.

> ## Box 6.2   Case law used to establish causation
>
> A widow made an attempt to claim that a doctor was negligent in not examining her husband in casualty who attended with arsenic poisoning and later died.
>
> The claim failed because the evidence proved that although the duty of care had been breached because he was not examined, if he had been seen and examined by a doctor, the outcome would still have been death.
>
> Hence, the cause of his death was not due to the breach in duty (Causation).
>
> Barnett v. Chelsea and Kensington Hospital Management Committee [1968] 1 All ER 1068.

To establish clinical negligence, a Court will ask a careful and responsible healthcare professional in similar role and circumstances how they would carry out the intervention or procedure in question. This was established from the case of *Bolam v. Friern Hospital Management Committee* [1957]. Mr Bolam underwent electroconvulsive therapy (ECT) to treat his depression but during the procedure, he sustained fractures due to fit-like convulsions that ECT can induce. He claimed that the doctor was negligent because he had not informed him of the risks or taken effective measures to prevent him from harm. The judge found the doctor not guilty of negligence for he acted:

in accordance with a practice accepted as proper by a responsible body of medical men skilled in that particular area" The test is the standard of the ordinary skilled man exercising and professing to have that special skill. A man need not possess the highest expert skill; it is well established law that it is sufficient if he exercises the ordinary skill of an ordinary competent man exercising that particular art. (Bolam v. Friern Hospital Management Committee [1957] 2 All ER118)

By seeking advice from other doctors who perform ECT, the Courts established that standard practice was consistent with those performing this intervention, therefore no negligence had occurred. This 'professional practice' standard or 'Bolam test' as it became known has been used to determine negligence for many years but was challenged in a later case of *Bolitho v. City and Hackney Health Authority* [1998] which questioned whether a judge should accept without question truthful evidence from eminent experts. Patrick Bolitho, aged 2, was admitted to hospital suffering from respiratory problems. A paediatric doctor was called on two occasions to attend the child but failed to do so. Patrick then suffered respiratory arrest leading to cardiac arrest causing catastrophic brain damage. The hospital admitted that the paediatric doctor had breached the duty of care by not attending but denied liability that the failure to attend had led to causation. The Bolam test was applied and the expert body of opinion for the claimant argued that Patrick should have been intubated; however, the expert body of opinion for the defendant felt that apart from the two episodes of respiratory distress, Patrick seemed generally well and because intubation involves risk for a young child, a responsible doctor would not have intubated the child. Reviewing precedent cases relating to claims of negligence against other professionals, the judge ruled that: The court has to be satisfied that the exponents of the body of opinion relied on can demonstrate that such opinion has a logical basis and

In cases of diagnosis and treatment there are cases where, despite a body of professional opinion sanctioning the defendants conduct, the defendant can properly be held liable for negligence because in some cases it cannot be demonstrated to the judges satisfaction that the body of opinion relied upon is reasonable and responsible. (Bolitho v. City and Hackney Health Authority [1998] AC 232)

This case demonstrates that courts are prepared to critically scrutinise the 'professional practice' standard. Therefore, for a negligence claim to succeed not only does a breach of duty and causation have to be established, the expert evidence from a person skilled in the same profession has to stand up to logical analysis by the Court. It endorsed judicial power to disregard expert testimony in exceptional cases.

Damages awarded for negligence are made up of a number of categories which takes into account not only physical harm but also psychiatric harm. It reflects real costs to the patient and not punishment for the defendant. Brazier and Cave (2007) inform that the patient's damages will be addressed to compensate for actual or prospective loss, loss of earnings, pain, suffering and disability which has been endured and will be endured in the future. The patient will be awarded the amount to cover extra expenses which the patient and family may incur.

An important way of ensuring that you do not carelessly harm a patient and avoid a potential litigation claim is to follow local and national policy, not to work beyond your competency, adhere to professional regulatory frameworks and to document every care intervention. This usually provides the practitioner with vicarious liability meaning that an employer becomes vicariously (indirectly) liable for negligence and any other wrongful acts or omissions of any employee acting in the course of employment providing professional standards and local policy have been followed.

Patient autonomy

The word autonomy is derived from the Greek 'autos' meaning 'self' and 'nomos' meaning 'rule', governance or law. Beauchamp and Childress (2008) note that autonomy has since been extended to individuals and has acquired meanings as diverse as self governance, liberty, rights, privacy, individual choice and freedom of will. Gillon (2005) advises that for a person to be autonomous, they must have the capacity to think, decide and act on the basis of such thought and decision freely and independently without hindrance. Patient autonomy now has important emphasis placed upon it and it is therefore common courtesy and a legal requirement that a healthcare professional not only respects patient autonomy but also ensures that a patient is not coerced into any unwanted treatment.

Consent to treatment

The law surrounding consent with so many diverse patient groups to take into consideration can often appear very daunting. Healthcare professionals need to be aware of the legalities surrounding consent to avoid litigation from non-consensual contact.

There are varying types of consent that can be obtained from patients. Tacit consent is expressed silently or passively by omissions, for example, if a patient lacked objection to a question, then this would constitute tacit consent. Implicit or implied consent can be inferred from actions either by a patient holding out their arm to have their blood pressure taken or allowing routine examination by their consultant in outpatients. Consent can be given verbally by a patient agreeing to treatment or in written form. Although the law in the United Kingdom acknowledges that patients should not be treated without consent to prevent legalities of assault and battery, there is no specific requirement that consent for treatment should be given in any particular way and any form of consent is valid. The exception is by Statute under the Mental Health Act 1983, the Human Fertilisation and Embryology Act 1990 or an advanced directive under the Mental Capacity Act 2005 which states that written consent is needed. It could be argued that unless written, other forms of consent are unsubstantial and it is professional guidance; local hospital policy and the Department of Health (DH) that suggest written consent ensure validity.

Informed consent

Patient consent has been an important ethical issue in the doctor–patient relationship for many years. According to Beauchamp and Childress (2008), from the early 1970s, the professional focus has shifted from the doctor's or researcher's obligation to disclose information to the patient's understanding of what they are giving consent for. This has introduced into practice a new term of 'informed consent'. The shift in emphasis has meant that doctors now have a professional and ethical obligation to their patient to ensure that when consent is obtained, the patient is sufficiently informed of the procedure being performed, any alternative treatment or potential risks, thus ensuring an autonomous consensual decision is given to accept, reject or seek an alternate treatment.

The patient should be informed in broad terms with as much information as a person feels they need to make choice and presented in a way that a person can understand with limited medical jargon; the inability to communicate needs to be addressed and the use of an interpreter for those where English is not their first language should be used. A claim of negligence could be sought if insufficient information is given by a doctor when obtaining patient consent to undergo treatment.

Montgomery (2003) states that the validity of patient consent depends upon a number of factors. In order to be valid, consent must be 'real'. Patients must be competent to give consent, must know what they are consenting to and must give their consent freely without being deliberately misled in order to arrive at their autonomous choice. Therefore, obtaining consent requires expertise, knowledge and advice from a professional and involves, shared care planning and decision making, to include the personal choice of the patient to accept or refuse their treatment. Common law recognises the principle that every competent person has the right to have bodily integrity protected against invasion by others which is also recognised within the 1951 European Convention on Human Rights, where article 9 states that everyone has the right to freedom of thought. The relevance of this regarding patient consent is that it is a fundamental human right for a patient to have autonomy when consenting to treatment. This ensures that procedures are performed ethically and legally, as the law views treatment without consent as an invasion of this self determination and integrity. However, due to ambiguity and the complexity of providing emergency treatment establishing whether a patient is making an informed autonomous decision can be problematic for paramedics due to many constraints, for example, anxiety, fear, alcohol or a range of medical conditions that can lead to confusion. It could be argued that these constraints not only impact on providing adequate patient care but also that practitioners could be in breach of their professional guidelines when establishing if patient consent is valid.

It is a fundamental human right that competent, autonomous adult patients with capacity have the right to refuse treatment. This also applies to a pregnant woman even if refusal threatens the life of her unborn child providing the woman has capacity when she refuses treatment. Refusal of treatment for those with capacity was established by Lord Donaldson in 1994 in the case of *Re C*. This case was that of a schizophrenic man detained in a mental hospital who refused to have his gangrenous leg amputated to save his life. His autonomous decision was to die with both his legs. His capacity was questioned and after much deliberation, the court ruling established a three-stage test (see Box 6.3) to determine whether he had the capacity to refuse treatment. Although this patient had his capacity questioned because he refused life-saving treatment, it highlights the need for patient choice, self determination and autonomy when making a decision. A choice to refuse treatment can appear irrational and uncomfortable to accept for the healthcare workers who are duty bound to beneficence and relieve suffering. It is considered by many patients that doctors know best but this case evidences that the patient's opinion and autonomous decision is also of importance. This case sets a precedent in English Law and evidences that any person can refuse life-saving medical intervention if they can satisfy doctors using the three stage 'Re C test' (see Box 6.3) that they have capacity.

Box 6.3   Three-stage test for refusal of treatment

If he could satisfy doctors that he could

● Comprehend and retain information
● Believe the information
● Weigh the information in the balance to arrive at a choice then, he was competent to make his decision to refuse life-saving treatment

RE C (Adult refusal of treatment) [1994] 1 All ER 819.

Paramedics will encounter difficulty obtaining consent for patients who are temporarily incapacitated, for example those who attend in a state of collapse and are temporarily unconscious, therefore unable to consent. Unless a lasting power of attorney (LPA) has been appointed in an advanced directive, friends, family and long term carers cannot give or withhold consent on behalf of anyone else. Patients who are incapacitated are treated using the best interest principle and the principle of necessity to provide life-saving treatment in urgent situations. This arises from a professional, objective paternalistic decision and duty of care to provide treatment that would be in the patient's best interests.

Consent for children

Attitudes towards children have changed dramatically over time. The rules around consent for minors younger than 16 years have been established from the case law of *Gillick v. West Norfolk and Wisbech Area Health Authority*

[1985]. The plaintiff, Mrs Gillick, had five daughters under the age of 16 and wanted assurance from her local health authority that her daughters would not be given contraception without Mrs Gillick being informed. The Health Authority would not give this assurance, so Mrs Gillick brought an action against the Health Authority. It was ruled in this case that

> *once a child under the age of 16 has sufficient understanding and intelligence to know what is involved in a proposed treatment he or she is defined as a 'Gillick competent minor' and can consent to therapeutic treatment. (Gillick v. West Norfolk and Wisbech Area Health Authority [1985])*

Paramedics will need to assess whether the mature minor is 'Gillick competent', therefore achieving the sufficient age, maturity and understanding to give consent for treatment. However, the Law does not recognise or give children under the age of 18 years the autonomy to refuse treatment and so consent must be given by those with parental responsibility unless the best interest principle is applied.

Confidentiality

Some of the most difficult dilemmas have arisen over the ethical obligation to protect patient confidentiality and privacy. This is without doubt the expectation of a patient when they enter into a relationship which requires divulging sensitive information about their health and social well-being. It is imperative to have a trustworthy and truth-telling relationship between the healthcare professionals and patient for the healthcare to be effective. The patient imparting the information binds the recipient to an obligation of confidence with the exception of divulging information to other team members to continue their care. Healthcare professionals not only have a professional duty to retain confidential information, it is a professional regulation and is often written into contracts of employment obliging the healthcare worker to keep all information confidential. Action will be taken if there is a breach of contract and disclosure of information which in turn could lead to disciplinary actions like termination of employment, loss of registration or Court action, if the patient decides to sue. Depending on the sensitivity of the disclosure, if suffering can be established there is little doubt that the tort of negligence could be upheld. It is imperative that healthcare workers remain diligent, not only during working hours but also off duty when conversing with family and friends in public areas.

Many statutes have been implemented to ensure the protection of confidentiality and privacy. The Data Protection Act 1998 imposes a duty upon organisations to promote the rights of patients and respect for the integrity of their medical records. It governs the storage, use and processing of personal data to ensure it conforms to the procedures laid out in the Act. The

Human Right Act 1998 provides protection for the rights of patients to privacy recognised in human rights Law where article 8 states that individuals have the right to respect for family private life. This emphasises the duty to protect the privacy of individuals and preserve confidentiality of their health records. Yet the nature of modern healthcare brings significant challenges to the management of confidential information. The increase of multidisciplinary teams and the introduction of NHS information technology mean that no longer do we have the patient–healthcare practitioner relationship with handwritten unseen records, but the electronic transmission of sensitive medical data which could potentially cause confidentiality to be inadvertently breached.

DH has played an important part in upholding patient confidentiality publishing guidance on protection and use of patient information and then implementing the Caldicott Report 1998. The Caldicott recommendations were to ensure patient identifiable information was transferred confidentially between organisations, the purpose for transfer was justified and only the minimum information necessary would be communicated. Protocols were to be developed to provide healthcare workers with guidance on sharing information across organisations, therefore being compliant with the Law. Caldicott guardians were put in place within healthcare organisations to ensure a confidential service was provided. Following on from the Caldicott Report, the DH published the NHS Confidentiality code of practice in 2003; this was introduced after major public consultation with patients, citizens, professional bodies and regulators of the NHS. It introduced the concept of confidentiality, provided a model of how a confidential service should be developed and the legal requirements for sharing information.

Information can be shared between healthcare professionals to provide treatment but in some situations, disclosure and use of confidential information is required by law and allowed without fear of litigation but it needs to be lawful and ethical. It is important that, where possible, patients are made aware and give their consent to disclose their information; however, the amount of information disclosed needs to be in proportion to the need required for the disclosure.

The Law requires disclosure of information in specific instances. The Public Health (Control of Disease) Act 1984 states that specified diseases are notifiable to the Health Authority allowing for lawful breaches of confidence to prevent the disease from spreading. However, this information can only be disclosed to medical practitioners or those employed under their direction. Acquired immunodeficiency syndrome (AIDS) or human immunodeficiency virus (HIV) is not a notifiable disease because although infectious, it is thought that by acting responsibly the infected person can reduce the risk to others, whereas disclosure could lead to an individual being afraid to seek treatment due to fear of a life of ridicule.

Information must also be disclosed if it leads to the identification of person involved in motor vehicle accident or to the Driving Vehicle Licence Agency if a person is deemed medically unfit to continue driving and needs to have their licence revoked.

Disclosure is also lawful if it is for the patient's best interests. For example when a paramedic is faced with an unconscious patient, discussion with a family member would require disclosure of information to enable the delivery of effective care. The DH (2003) states that if a patient is unconscious or unable, due to a mental or physical condition, to give consent or to communicate a decision, the health professionals concerned must take decisions about the use of information.

In situations where a patient may put the public at risk, an obligation arises to protect the well-being of the community, so disclosure is required in public interest to prevent harm. Brazier and Cave (2007) inform that personal information may be disclosed in public interest without patient consent where the benefits to an individual or to society of the disclosure outweigh the public and patient's interests in keeping confidential information. The HCPC (2012d) suggests considering the possible risk of harm to other people when deciding to breach confidential information in public interest and to speak to your employer or seek legal advice. They recommend keeping clear records as you may be asked to justify your decision.

Confidentiality for minors

The House of Lords not only endorsed in the case of *Gillick v. West Norfolk and Wisbech*[1985] that a child under the age of 16 with sufficient knowledge, understanding and intelligence to know what is involved in their treatment can give autonomous consent. This case also endorsed that a doctor owes a duty of confidentiality to a patient less than 16 years of age if they have capacity and understanding to take decisions about their treatment. Therefore, the precedent 'Gillick' case ruled that in exceptional cases the doctor is free to treat a minor without parental knowledge if they have the capacity, competence and maturity to consent to treatment.

Mental health and mental capacity

The MHA 1983 and its amendments in the 2007 Mental Health Act regulates mental healthcare and legalises the compulsory detention for assessment and treatment of certain people with a mental disorder which threatens their health or safety or the safety of the public. The Mental Health Act Commission oversees the implementation of these Acts and ensures the protection and safeguarding of patients' rights. The Mental Health Act was amended in 2007 because the 1983 Act was outdated due to the fact that mental health has moved away from the large hospitals using the institutional approach that were around in the 1980s and moved more into providing community care where possible. It provides a statutory framework to protect those who lack capacity and covers decisions not already provided for by the 1983 MHA. These Acts of Parliament are concerned with the circumstances in which a person with a mental illness can be detained for treatment for their disorder without consent. It also sets the processes that must be followed and the safeguards for the patient to ensure they are not inappropriately detained or treated without their consent.

When a person is said to be 'sectioned', the terminology arises from the sections from the Mental Health Act that allows for lawful non-consensual detainment. Section 2 of the MHA 1983 states that a person may be detained for assessment and treatment for up to 28 days if they suffer from a mental disorder. Section 3 states that a person can be detained for treatment for up to 6 months and this period can be renewed if the patient is suffering from mental illness, psychopathic disorder or mental impairment which requires medical treatment. People can only be detained under the MHA 1983 if they become aggressive or demonstrate seriously irresponsible conduct, therefore a person with severe learning disability cannot be detained. It must be emphasised that non-consensual detainment is for the treatment and assessment of mental health only.

An approved social worker or the person's nearest relative can make an application for detainment but two medical practitioners must support the application. To consider a formal admission under the MHA 1983, an Approved Mental Health professional (AMHP) has to certify that the patient is suffering from a mental disorder and compulsory detainment is necessary. The accountability lies with three key people, the AMHP who could be a local authority approved nurse or social worker with the competence to assess a mental disorder, a registered medical practitioner who is approved by the primary care trusts as competent to diagnose a mental disorder and the patient's relative. The patient has the right to appeal but cannot discharge themselves because they are detained by law under Section 2 or 3.

Under Section 135, a Magistrate can issue a warrant to allow a police officer to enter and remove a person by force if necessary if they suspect a person is suffering from a mental disorder, is being ill-treated, neglected, kept under improper control or they have gone absent under a compulsory Section 2 detention. This will allow the person to be returned to a place of safety. The police officer may be accompanied by a doctor or any person authorised to take the patient. Section 136 gives the police authority to remove people from a public place who appear to be suffering from a mental disorder and take them to a place of safety. The person can be detained for a maximum of 72 hours for examination by a doctor or interview by an AMHP.

Compulsory detention means that a person becomes deprived of their liberty; however, in recent years, case law has raised the issues of respecting autonomy and liberty for patients with a mental health disability. Changes became necessary after a case (*R v. Bournewood Community and Mental Health NHS Trust* [1998] 3 All ER 289) concerning an autistic man with profound learning disabilities who had lived in Bournewood Hospital from the age of 13. After 30 years he was discharged into the foster care to live in the community. After becoming agitated and distressed in a day centre, he was subsequently taken to the A&E department at Bournewood Hospital, sedated and detained under the Mental Health Act. His foster carers were not permitted to visit in case he became more distressed and attempted to leave with them. The foster carers applied to the Court to have this decision upturned. The judge ruled

> *that a man who had been informally admitted to a psychiatric hospital without capable consent had not been unlawfully detained under the common law. (R v Bournewood Community and Mental Health NHS Trust* [1998] 3 All ER 289)

However, an appeal later ruled in the European Court of Human Rights, that he had been unlawfully deprived of his liberty under the Article 5 of the European Convention on Human Rights. Following this, the government launched a widespread consultation about the potential consequences of 'the Bournewood judgment', as it became known to establish whether incapacitated adults in care homes, and hospitals were being deprived of their liberty. This consultation resulted in the amendment of the Mental Capacity Act 2005 to contain the 'deprivation of liberty safeguards' (DOLs). These safeguards provide administrative and judicial protection for adults who lack mental capacity to prevent arbitrary decisions that may deprive vulnerable people of their liberty. Everything that is done for a patient is to be in their best interest with the least restrictive intervention of their rights and freedoms.

Mental Capacity Act

The Mental Capacity Act received royal assent in 2005 but did not come into force until 2007. It provides statutory protection with clear safeguards to empower and protect vulnerable people who are not able to make their own decisions if they lose capacity. This will enable people to plan ahead for a time when they become incompetent. Validating a signed advanced directive will allow a person to nominate a proxy decision maker called an LPA to make decisions about their care, and makes clear who can make health and welfare decisions on their behalf and in which situations. This could lead to an area of uncertainty as a paramedic not only has to ensure that the advanced directive was made by the person when they had the capacity but also it must make clear that the treatment being refused. If a validated advanced directive cannot be produced, the paramedic will have to treat the patient using the best interest principle.

The LPA must be nominated whilst the patient has capacity and is registered with the Office of Public Guardian, and can only take control of decision making when the patient loses capacity. If there has not been a nominated power of attorney, then the Court of Protection could appoint a deputy to make personal and welfare decisions if they were satisfied that a deputy could fulfil the role.

As previously discussed, all patients have a right to make an autonomous decision providing they have capacity. If the decision to refuse treatment appears unwise, then this is not a reason for a healthcare professional to question a patient's capacity. The Mental Capacity Act 2005 sets out five principles in the code of practice and these values form the basis of the legal requirements in the act and a paramedic should familiarise themselves with this code of practice (see Box 6.4). In an emergency situation when a patient may present in a state of collapse or unconscious, urgent life-saving decisions have to be made by a paramedic. In this situation, the paramedic cannot delay treatment and will have no time to establish whether there is an LPA so will take action and provide treatment in the patient's best interests.

Box 6.4   The five principles of the Mental Capacity Act

1. A person must be assumed to have capacity unless it is established that they lack capacity.
2. A person is not to be treated as unable to make a decision unless all practicable steps to help him to do so have been taken without success.
3. A person is not to be treated as unable to make a decision merely because he makes an unwise decision.
4. An act done, or decision made, under this Act for or on behalf of a person who lacks capacity must be done, or made, in his best interests.
5. Before the act is done, or the decision is made, regard must be had to whether the purpose for which it is needed can be as effectively achieved in a way that is less restrictive of the person's rights and freedom of action.

Mental Capacity Act 2005 Code of Practice. The Stationery Office, London.

Ethical theories

The emergency quick decision making required by a paramedic to treat a patient leads to the paramedic being more vulnerable than other healthcare professionals when trying to respect their patient's wishes. It is therefore of paramount importance that they comprehend the ethical issues that will be encountered on a daily basis.

Ethical and moral reasoning is a fundamental part of the patient care decision-making process and shapes our professional codes. It is necessary when practitioners are confronted with awkward dilemmas within our multicultural world. Medical ethics and moral philosophy attempts to unravel the rights and wrongs of different areas of healthcare practice using philosophical analysis to ask questions about values, rights and wrongs and what ought or ought not to be done in a given situation. Within a society with such varied cultural beliefs, a practitioner must ensure that their own moral standards do not conflict with their patients requests and that the patient's best interests are put first to avoid imposing one's own moral code onto a patient.

Morality refers to norms and expectations that govern our beliefs about the right and wrong of human conduct and are so widely shared that they form a stable social consensus of what we owe to each other. Virtually everyone who grows up has a basic understanding of the institution of morality and its norms are readily understood, for example do not kill, keep promises, do not steal or do not tell lies. Moral choices are conditioned by our race, culture and education; they are not fixed and may vary between one group or society to another. All morals can be justifiably overridden; for example breaking promises or telling 'little white lies' to save hurting someone's feelings does not necessarily make someone immoral.

The Law however differs to morals and ethics in that it concerns the Courts and Parliament and is either something that is laid down explicitly in statute which comes into force at a specific date and time or from regulations or precedent cases; whereas moral judgements are not time bound. Both law and morality may contain many norms that are identical in content for example, the Law states do not kill and moral norms tell us this is wrong. However, it would be extremely difficult to legally regulate immoral issues and attempting to enforce the law would be unfeasible. The Law does have to play its part to enforce and govern morality if there could be harm to society. An example of this was the introduction of the Human Fertilisation and Embryology Act 1990. This statute arose after new technology made it possible for the first in vitro fertilisation (IVF) baby to be born in 1978. The government brought together a committee headed by a philosopher (Mary Warnock) to look into this controversial emotive issue and to regulate human embryo research.

Ethical enquiry is a complex process which is triggered when health professionals, patients and clients are faced with ethical issues and dilemmas in practice. It is not solely based on morals but also with the use of law, professional codes, social convention, religious codes and politics to support a moral judgement of what is right and wrong. Ethical judgements are perhaps the most difficult and unclear to make, so ethical theories are used to find some moral standard or rule to arrive at a decision.

Consequentialism

A consequentialist theory regards the right action in any situation to be the action that produces the best available consequence, thus acting to maximise good. Decisions can be calculated by weighing up the most good achieved by the various options. The consequence of an action is right if it produces most pleasure and the action is wrong if it produces suffering. However, an objection to consequentialism is that it could allow for horrific acts to be accepted, for example torturing someone for information if the overall outcome of the torture provided greater happiness for a greater number. This could make nothing unthinkable which morally we would need to question. It can also be very difficult to identify how people interpret and understand happiness and an empirical calculation would be needed to enable us to determine how to maximise good.

Utilitarianism

One of the most popular and dominant forms of consequentialism is utilitarianism. Utilitarian ethics was formulated first by Jeremy Bentham in 1781 and later developed further by the philosopher John Stuart Mill. Utilitarianism promotes one basic principle of ethics: the principle of utility and that the value of the consequences are measured by the 'greatest happiness principle' which suggests that each person's happiness counts for exactly the same as every others and that the value of an action is positive if and only if that action increases total happiness in the world. This principle is seen when a patient is refused an expensive cancer treatment which appears extremely unjust for the patient and family who are refused the treatment but applying this ethical theory and refusing an expensive drug to one patient would enable utilisation of limited NHS recourses to more patients with a better life expectancy, thus maximising good.

Deontology

Immanuel Kant first recognised this ethical theory in the late eighteenth century. Deontological moral theories coincide with consequentialism as they determine the action itself as the key to the rightness or wrongness and the outcome is determined by the action itself rather than by its consequence which should conform to a moral rule or principle. An example of this is the doctrine of double effect that is applied within medicine. This principle allows for the legal administration of large doses of morphine to relieve pain. The intended good primary action is to relive pain; however, the unintended second action due to the large doses of morphine being administered is respiratory depression leading to the speed up and onset of death.

Despite the differences between consequentialism and deontology, they share several common characteristics; both focus on actions or outcomes of actions, both structure around the concepts of right and wrong, good or bad. Consequentialism looks at the outcome whereas deontology looks at the act. However, tired of the consequentialism versus deontology debate, modern ethicists came up with the moral theory of principlism which consists of four principles. These principles provide a framework for reflecting and identifying moral problems giving guidance based on four principles to respect autonomy, non-maleficence (cause no harm), beneficence (provide benefit) and justice having an obligation to provide fairness in the distribution of benefits and risks (see also Chapter 7). Applying ethical theories and moral reasoning to difficult situations encountered by healthcare practitioners can enable decision making to be made.

Do not attempt resuscitation

An area in healthcare that often questions ethical decision making and can lead to conflict between patients, relatives and practitioners is when 'do not attempt resuscitation' (DNAR) orders are placed upon patients. It is of utmost importance to include the patient if possible and the family with the end of life decision-making process and to have clear policies and guidelines in place. The decision must be taken on an individual patient basis and local trusts will have clear protocols to guide a practitioner to recognise a valid DNAR order. Paramedics who often get called to patients at the end of their life need to deliver care with the utmost compassion and respect. They are often faced with huge ethical dilemmas regarding DNAR and could encounter conflict where family members disagree with the DNAR order and insist that resuscitation attempts commence or when the DNAR documentation is not readily available. In this situation, resuscitation must begin but can be withdrawn when the documentation confirms that a DNAR order has been arranged.

Summary

This chapter has provided an insight into the need for registration of healthcare professionals who need to have an understanding of their regulatory framework as they are accountable in ensuring they deliver effective patient care. Having a duty of care to their patients means that healthcare professionals must participate with CPD, adhere to their regulatory guidelines, scope of practice, national and local policy to provide protection of vicarious liability and avoid litigation and claims of negligence.

The vagueness and complexity of the law means that professional, legal and ethical issues can be confusing for healthcare professionals but having discussed case law, statutes and regulatory frameworks to protect both patient confidentiality and patient autonomy when obtaining consent, it has highlighted that keeping patient information confidential and respecting patient autonomy is a fundamental human right.

Analysis of the law for those that lack capacity to ensure that they are not deprived of their liberty and how advanced directives can be utilised under the Mental Capacity Act 2005 to refuse treatment by nominating an LPA to make decisions, now allows a patient the choice to plan ahead for a time when they are no longer competent. It was identified that paramedics frequently face the need for quick decision making at the end of a patient's life and can experience conflict where an advanced directive or DNAR order is unavailable.

The chapter concluded with discussion of how ethical theories and moral reasoning is used as part of the patient care decision-making process to resolve ethical dilemmas and how within a multi-cultural society, a practitioner must ensure that their own moral standards do not conflict with their patients' requests and that the patients' best interests are put first.

References

Beauchamp, T.L. & Childress, J.F. (2008) *Principles of Biomedical Ethics*, 6th edn. Oxford University Press, New York.

Brazier, M. & Cave, E. (2007) *Medicines, Patients and the Law*, 4th edn. Penguin, London.

Department of Health (DH) (2003) *Confidentiality. NHS Code of Practice*. Department of Health, London.

Gillon, R. (2005) *Philosophical Medical Ethics*. John Wiley & Sons, Chichester.

Health & Care Professions Council (HCPC) (2012a) *Standards of Conduct, Performance and Ethics*. HCPC, London.

Health & Care Professions Council (HCPC) (2012b) *We have changed our name*. Available at http://www.hpc-uk.org/aboutus/namechange/ (accessed 10 August 2012).

Health & Care Professions Council (HCPC) (2012c) *Standards of Proficiency. Paramedic*. HCPC, London.

Health & Care Professions Council (HCPC) (2012d) *Confidentiality-Guidance for Registrants*. HCPC, London.

Health & Care Professions Council (HCPC) (2012e) *Your Guide to Our Standards for Continuing Professional Development*. HCPC, London.

Joint Royal College Ambulance Liaison Committee (2006) *UK Ambulance Service Clinical Practice Guidelines*. Available at http://www2.warwick.ac.uk/

fac/med/research/hsri/emergencycare/prehospitalcare/jrcalcstakeholder
website/guidelines/clinical_guidelines_2006.pdf (accessed May 2012).

Mason, J. & McCall Smith, R. (2011) *Law and Medical Ethics*, 8th edn. Oxford
University Press, New York.

McHale, J. & Fox, M. (2007) *Healthcare Law*, 2nd edn. Sweet & Maxwell, London.

Mental Capacity Act (2005) *Code of Practice*. The Stationery Office, London.

Montgomery, J. (2003) *Health Care Law*, 2nd edn. Oxford University Press, Oxford.

National Health Service Litigation Authority (NHSLA) (2011) *The National
Health Service Litigation Authority. Reports and Accounts 2010–11*. Available at
http://www.nhsla.com/AboutUs/Documents/NHSLA Annual Report and
Accounts 2011.pdf (accessed March 2012).

National Health Service Litigation Authority [NHSLA] (2012) *NHSLA
Risk Management Standards for Ambulance Services 2012–13*. Available
at http://www.nhsla.com/Safety/Documents/NHSLA Risk Management
Standards 2012 13 for Ambulance Services.pdf (accessed March 2012).

Case Law

Barnett v. Chelsea and Kensington Hospital Management Committee [1968]
1 All ER 1068.

Bolam v. Friern Hospital Management Committee [1957] 2 All ER 118.

Bolitho v. City and Hackney Health Authority [1998] AC 232.

Gillick v. West Norfolk and Wisbech [1985] 3 All ER 402.

RE C (Adult refusal of treatment) [1994] 1 All ER 819.

R v. Bournewood Community and Mental Health NHS Trust [1998] 3 All ER
289.

Table of Statutes

Caldicott Report 1998.

Data Protection Act 1998.

European Convention on Human Rights 1951.

Health Professions Order 2001.

Human Fertilisation and Embryology Act 1990.

Human Right Act 1998.

Mental Capacity Act 2005.

Mental Health Act [MHA] 1983.

Mental Health Act [MHA] 2007.

Public Health (Control of Disease) Act 1984.

NHS Redress Act 2006.

Public Interest Disclosure Act 1998.

7 Anti-discriminatory Practice

Matt Capsey

School of Health and Social Care, Teesside University, Middlesbrough, UK

Introduction

The notion of anti-discriminatory practice arises in several places within contemporary paramedic education and practice. It is a Health & Care Professions Council (HCPC) requirement within paramedics' standards of proficiency (HCPC, 2012) and the Quality Assurance Agency (QAA) highlight it within the benchmarks for paramedic science programmes (QAA, 2004). The term, however, remains poorly defined between professions and can conjure up negative connotations. This chapter will look at the development of anti-discriminatory practice from its roots in social work theory through its adoption by wider health and social care. To practise in an anti-discriminatory or culturally competent way requires a basic understanding of discrimination from its basis in cognitive processes through the formation of prejudices and potentially onto oppression.

Having established a brief introduction to discrimination, the ethical and legal basis of anti-discriminatory practice will be considered, including the requirements of the HCPC and various Acts of Parliament. These Acts form a practical basis on which to define discrimination as it may appear in paramedic practice, positive or negative, direct or indirect. Whilst the focus of this chapter will be paramedic practice in the United Kingdom, it is equally applicable to others working in pre-hospital and wider healthcare. There are more similarities between arbitrarily defined groups than the perceived differences and this applies to healthcare job titles as much as ethnic groups and this shall also be included. An understanding of the theoretical basis is not enough and paramedics must be self-aware and able to challenge their own practice to ensure it meets the highest standards.

The second half of the chapter will revisit the cognitive basis of discrimination and prejudice, look at how equality and diversity can be supported and how the skills for cultural competency can be developed. It is outside the scope of this chapter to identify all the subtleties and intricacies

Professional Practice in Paramedic, Emergency and Urgent Care, First Edition. Edited by Val Nixon.
© 2013 John Wiley & Sons, Ltd. Published 2013 by John Wiley & Sons, Ltd.

of the United Kingdom's vast cultural mix, in fact to try and create a mental catalogue such as this would be counterproductive for the paramedic. The United Kingdom has always contained significant numbers of migrant groups. These are constantly changing and vary in their visibility within the general population. When thinking initially about discrimination or cultural competence many readers may be drawn to groups that appear visibly different; however, it would be a mistake to assume that it is only visible minorities that suffer discrimination. Examples given through the chapter aim to highlight some of the many groups, usually (though not always) minority groups, that continue to experience discrimination in the United Kingdom today.

Most proficient paramedics will be working in an anti-discriminatory manner and it is useful that the usual one-to-one nature of their practice lends itself to enhance their skills. By the end of this chapter it is hoped that the reader will have a more detailed understanding of discrimination and is able to interrogate and reflect on their own thoughts and feelings to ensure that their practice never knowingly or unwittingly contributes to the continued discrimination of any group in society.

Definitions and theory of anti-discriminatory practice

Anti-discriminatory practice is an approach to the provision of health and social care that emerged from social work theory during the 1980s. Prior to the adoption of anti-discriminatory practice, social work (and healthcare) focused on addressing the needs of individual clients rather than placing them in their social context and acting to change it. Without addressing their context, it was difficult to address the many challenges faced by clients that have their roots outside of the individual, and consequently these would continue to affect both the client and others in similar circumstances. Since the difficulties that their clients faced may have been due to discrimination by outside organisations and wider society, there was a shift in social work practice to challenge, mitigate and, wherever possible, remove the sources of discrimination that were affecting clients and their wider social group. This approach became widely adopted in social work and its benefits are now recognised as a guiding principle not only in social work but in wider healthcare and other public services and organisations.

When treating a patient who is valued as an individual, it is not acceptable to only address their clinical need without any thought to the context within which they experience their life. How professionals practice in an anti-discriminatory manner varies but all seek to place the patient, client or service user's needs at the centre of care. They recognise that not all of these needs have their roots within the individual but some may arise from discrimination against that individual or the manner in which services are organised that creates a barrier to access. Personal discrimination and any discrimination caused by service organisation are unacceptable and should be removed.

Before we can begin to practise in an anti-discriminatory manner, we must first understand the nature of the discrimination we are seeking to remove. It would be too simplistic to assert that we should not discriminate at all in the way we treat patients. It is a necessary and wholly appropriate part of any caring profession to recognise the differences between patients and treat them accordingly. Processes such as triage and care planning look to discriminate between patients' needs and assign resources and treatment appropriately. Neil Thompson, one of the key writers on anti-discriminatory practice, has recognised that the literal sense of discrimination is *to detect difference*. He sees that to diminish the importance of anti-discriminatory practice on the grounds of narrow semantics is to miss the profound effect discrimination and oppression has on those who experience them (Thompson *cited in* Scullion, 2000). The nature of discrimination that requires challenge is based on individual characteristics of patients not immediately linked to their clinical needs such as their age, gender, ethnicity, education level or socio-economic class. At this point, it may be useful to consider the psychological basis of discrimination and the difference that Thompson (2005) identifies between simple discrimination and that leads to prejudice and oppression.

As stated above, in its most basic form, discrimination is the detection of difference. Effective paramedic practice requires the ability to discriminate between patterns of symptoms to reach a working diagnosis and plan the ongoing care of a patient. In a multiple casualty incident, it is necessary to be able to quickly discriminate between patient's clinical circumstances to ensure that limited resources are targeted at those most in need. With practice, this decision making becomes easier as many of our cognitive processes have evolved around pattern recognition and the identification of similarity and difference. Unfortunately, these same cognitive processes, that allow rapid decision making in complex situations, also create the basis of stereotyping, prejudice and discrimination.

As social animals, humans tend to form themselves into groups and define themselves in terms of that group, be it sporting teams, occupations, gender or nationality. In an effort to promote intragroup cohesiveness and identity, we have a tendency to emphasise the similarities between the members of our group (the *in-group*). Additionally, we also tend to emphasise the differences between ourselves and others outside our group (the *out-group*). As an example of these tendencies, political parties can provide a good example: Parties will tend to describe themselves in broad terms such as 'low taxation', 'pro-union', 'anti-immigration', 'pro-European' and seek to portray opposition parties as taking up a contrary position. They seek to present a united front in an effort to gain votes and win political power; however, when questioned in detail, individual members can be seen to have very wide views on each policy area. There can be a wider difference in individuals' views within each party than there is between parties' official stances, to the point where on the periphery individuals from different parties can hold almost identical views. So it is with any other arbitrary grouping such as ethnicity, religion or even gender.

Within practice, it is important to ensure that patients are treated as individuals and arbitrary characteristics are not attributed due to their group identity, either positively for members of an *in-group* or negatively for members of an *out-group*. At this point, it should be said that there are occasions when making assumptions based on group membership may be valid but opportunities should be sought to challenge them. As an example, in a patient of Afro-Caribbean appearance suffering difficulty in breathing and joint pain, a working diagnosis of sickle cell crisis may be reasonable; however, the paramedic must remain open to alternative diagnoses for this patient; similarly, another patient with the same symptoms but of Northern European appearance should not have the diagnosis of sickle cell crisis ruled out on the basis of their physical appearance alone.

Where simple discrimination is the process of recognising the different characteristics of things or people, for example, their size, shape or colour, it can move onto become prejudice when values are attached to those characteristics (e.g. big hands are nicer than small hands) or other unrelated characteristics are linked to the perceived difference (e.g. people with big hands are less intelligent). When presented in these terms, prejudice can appear almost comical, however, its invidious nature should not be underestimated. It becomes a wholly more serious issue when there is a power imbalance associated with it, giving the opportunity for one individual or group to disadvantage another on the basis of their prejudices. In the presence of a power imbalance, discrimination can move from prejudice into the realms of oppression. Despite all best efforts there will always be a power imbalance between a clinician and their patient. Actively seeking to reduce that imbalance, by empowering the patient wherever possible to be involved in their care, can reduce the risk of discriminatory practice. Paramedics must ensure that they do not, either unintentionally or intentionally, reduce the quality of the care provided to any patient due to that power imbalance. Many patients will have experienced discrimination throughout their lives and it is important that paramedics do not reinforce that discrimination but instead support them to overcome it.

This is the negative form of discrimination that anti-discriminatory practice seeks to challenge and undermine. It should therefore be obvious that it is this form of discrimination that is being referred to throughout the rest of the chapter rather than the simpler categorisation. The precise definitions of discrimination and oppression in the context of paramedic practice will be discussed later.

Discussion point

Think about a group you have little contact with, possibly ethnic but may be national or even geographic. What are the differences between you and the members of this group and what are the similarities? Now, think carefully how you came to those decisions, what are they based on? If you have little contact are you basing your ideas on a limited number of individuals that you have met, or on images you have seen in the media? How reliable are these as sources of information and what are the potential consequences for your care when dealing with a member of this group?

Ethical and legal basis of anti-discriminatory practice

Anti-discriminatory practice arises from the basic ethical principles that govern all healthcare practice. The models developed by Beauchamp and Childress (1977), and Iserson et al. (1995) serve to illustrate that discrimination on anything other than clinical grounds is unethical. Since its first publication in 1977, Beauchamp and Childress's work has remained one of the key influences in medical ethics. They provide four key areas: autonomy, beneficence, non-maleficence and justice (Beauchamp and Childress, 2001). Respect for autonomy requires that the patient is placed at the centre of their care. To the modern reader, this may appear almost too obvious to require stating. However, historically the medical establishment was seen as having a very paternalistic approach to patients; acting as though the health professional knows best and the patient's role is to do as they are told. It has taken concerted effort to move to patient-centred care and a wise paramedic should not assume that everyone else shares their commitment to respect the patient's autonomy. Including patients in their care should be the goal of all paramedics and only be overridden when to do so is clearly impractical.

Beneficence requires that paramedics should act in the patient's best interest and all actions should be focused on either improving their condition or helping them with the situation in which they find themselves. For the help available to be given or withheld based on a patient's gender, socio-economic class or some other arbitrary aspect of their identity rather than clinical need would be clearly wrong. Discriminating against a patient, for example, withholding treatment based on their age, may cause them clinical harm, is not in their best interest and as such goes contrary to the principle of non-maleficence, commonly referred to as 'first do no harm'. Beauchamp and Childress's (2001) fourth aspect of justice is most clearly linked to anti-discriminatory practice. It reflects the ethical position of universalism in that the interventions used or treatment given should be the same in all equal situations. It does not preclude the rationing of health-care; however, all patients should have fair access to the available resources and where priorities need to be set they should not be to the disadvantage of one or more groups.

Beauchamp and Childress's (2001) framework for ethical practice can at times seem removed from the everyday practicalities of delivering health-care in the paramedic environment. An approach more closely designed to meet the needs of emergency medicine is the framework proposed by Iserson et al. (1995) for making rapid ethically sound decisions. When a situation is time critical and there is no current rule (law, protocol or guide-line), they suggest the professionals should ask themselves three questions when deciding on a course of action:

- Would you be willing to have this action performed if you were the patient?
- Would you be willing to use the same solution in any similar cases?
- Would you be willing to defend the decision to others, and to share the decision in public?

From these questions, it is clear that to base a decision in these circum-stances on a patient's physical appearance, class, religion or any other ar-bitrary characteristic would be untenable.

Law and ethics are not synonymous; however, they are closely linked. When a society has developed clear ethical standpoints these often become enshrined in law. Anti-discriminatory practice is one such area and it has led to specific laws and contributed to other legislation. To practise in the United Kingdom, paramedics are required to be registered with the HCPC; this was enshrined in law in the Health Profession Order 2001. To remain registered, paramedics must adhere to the HCPC's (2012) Standards of Pro-ficiency. These include the following:

1a.1   Be able to practise within the legal and ethical boundaries of their profession.
- Understand the need to act in the best interests of service users at all times.
- Understand the need to respect, and so far as possible uphold, the rights, dignity, values and autonomy of every service user . . .
1a.2   Be able to practise in a non-discriminatory manner.
1b.3   Be able to demonstrate effective and appropriate skills in communi-cating information, advice, instruction and professional opinion to colleagues, service users, their relatives and carers.
- Be aware of the characteristics and consequences of non-verbal communication and how this can be affected by culture, age, eth-nicity, gender, religious beliefs and socio-economic status.

- Recognise that relationships with service users should be based on mutual respect and trust, and be able to maintain high standards of care even in situations of personal incompatibility.

Outside of their professional registration, paramedics must also meet the requirements of several legal Acts related to discrimination. It is outside the scope of this chapter to list in detail all of these Acts; however, the key ones include the Mental Capacity Act 2005, Sex Discrimination Act 1975, Race Relations (Amendment) Act 2000, Disability Discrimination Act 2005 and the Equality Act 2010. The Mental Capacity Act 2005 was not drafted specifically to address discrimination; however, it has that effect in its requirements to be mindful of the wishes of those who lack capacity. This can be seen to work against discrimination directed against those with a mental or cognitive disability, a physical disability that affects the communication of their decisions or arguably discrimination on the grounds of age for those suffering dementia. In 2010, the Equality Act repealed and replaced four previous Acts: the Equal Pay Act 1970, Sex Discrimination Act 1975, Race Relations (Amendment) Act 2000 and Disability Discrimination Act 2005, along with three statutory instruments. The 2010 Equality Act identifies nine protected characteristics which is unlawful to discriminate on the grounds of (with a few exceptions). These protected characteristics are age, disability, gender reassignment, marriage and civil partnership, pregnancy and maternity, race, religion or belief, sex and sexual orientation. These will be looked at in more detail later in the chapter. It also identifies the ways in which it is unlawful to treat an individual including both direct and indirect discrimination, failing to make a reasonable adjustment for a disabled person, harassment and victimisation.

Chapter 6 discusses additional legislative and professional requirements in more detail.

Definitions of discrimination and oppression

Discrimination

It has been established earlier that discrimination refers to the treatment of an individual less favourably on the grounds of their membership of a group or an identifying characteristic rather than on that individual's merit and is defined as such in the Equality Act 2010. Discrimination may be positive or negative; however, within a healthcare setting, especially in the United Kingdom where health provision has historically been allocated on a patient's need, it is never acceptable to base treatment decisions on a discriminatory approach. At first glance, this appears to be self-evident and few paramedics would consider themselves as being discriminatory in their practice, nevertheless the nature of discrimination is such that it may occur due to the nature of how services are provided or due to unconscious stereotypes held by the individual. The process of reducing discrimination against one group may paradoxically increase discrimination against another. For example, where financial resources are limited, the introduction of an outreach clinic for one minority group may lead to a reduction in resources for translation services for another.

Anti-discriminatory practice seeks to consciously look for occasions where discrimination may occur and ensure that there are strategies in place to prevent or minimise these opportunities. Within a large organisation, this would include having policies on discrimination and ensuring that the staff are regularly updated in line with current best practice on equality and diversity. At the level of the individual paramedic, it is important to be self-aware. The paramedic should reflect on the potential prejudices they hold and aim to minimise them, ensuring they are aware of the support available and have strategies to deal with situations where discrimination may occur. The first step to minimise one's own prejudices is to recognise what they are. As previously identified, prejudice can come from subconsciously comparing one's own identifying characteristics to others'. To be self-aware, paramedics should be aware of their own culture and ethnicity. Defining one's own culture can be very challenging, as can facing up to the reality of your own biases and prejudices. However, without this self-knowledge it is not possible to be culturally competent or effectively challenge discrimination by other individuals or organisations.

Negative discrimination

The discrimination considered up to this point could all be described as negative discrimination. Most of the examples given are related to direct, overt discrimination. A clear example of an overtly negative discriminatory practice would be specifying in a job advert that applicant must be male. However, some negative discrimination is more subtle being indirect or covert, such as when provision is lacking for a certain group: an imbalance in single sex accommodation, literature not being available in formats for those with a visual impairment or a requirement that patients give a home address prior to treatment (this would discriminate against the homeless) (see also Box 7.1).

Box 7.1   Example of positive discrimination

An ambulance service introduces a partnership with schools in an area of socio-economic deprivation. They provide talks to pupils and work experience placements to demonstrate that the paramedic profession is a realistic goal for local children. The long term goal of the intervention is to ensure that applicants from this area stand as good a chance as those from more privileged backgrounds when applying for paramedic training and eventually changing the profile of the workforce to better reflect the local community.

Positive discrimination

Positive discrimination exists where (usually) underrepresented groups are sought out and given preferential treatment over others. This is most usually seen within recruitment as employers seek to balance their workforce by employing more women or individuals from specific ethnic minorities. Positive discrimination can lead onto negative discrimination against either the current dominant group or other minority groups not directly targeted. An advert that positively discriminates by requesting an Asian applicant would be negatively discriminating against black applicants or those from a Romany background, groups which may also be underrepresented.

Under current UK law, *positive discrimination* is illegal in employment practices; however, NHS trusts may engage in *positive action* to address inequalities in opportunity. NHS employers (2005, p. 1) defined positive action as:

> A range of lawful actions that seeks to address an imbalance in employment opportunities among targeted groups that have previously experienced disadvantage, or that have been subject to discriminatory policies and practices, or that are underrepresented in the workforce.

They are clear that the recruitment process must select the candidate most suited to the job in question. Positive action comprises a range of methods to prepare disadvantaged groups for the recruitment process (see example in Box 7.2). These may include work experience placements, personal mentoring or assistance in accessing qualifications.

Box 7.2   Example of negative discrimination

Due to the increasing number of bariatric patients, an ambulance service introduces an employment requirement that employees must be able to lift a certain weight. At first glance, this appears neutral and intended to ensure patient safety. However, it is indirectly discriminatory against women. Whilst any individual candidate, of either gender, may or may not achieve the target, there will be more women who fail to meet the requirement than men. Therefore, to be anti-discriminatory in ensuring the safety of bariatric patients, the service chooses to introduce extra patient handling and lifting equipment.

Outside of employment issues and of equal interest to paramedics, the NHS runs many schemes that seek to positively discriminate in favour of certain groups. Much has been written about health inequalities across the United Kingdom and various health screening programmes have been set up to address them. In 2009, the Parliamentary Health Select Committee (HSC) identified that addressing health inequalities should pervade everything from health promotion to specialist services. In the wider NHS schemes that positively discriminate in favour of certain groups include screening programmes for older people and the setting up of clinics or outreach projects for traveller and Gypsy communities, a group who have demonstrably lower health outcomes than the fixed population (Parry et al., 2007). Since positive discrimination is illegal under the Equality Act 2010 and positive action is accomplished at an organisational level, there may appear to be little that the operational paramedic does related to positive discrimination. However, there is an expectation that minority groups should expect the same level of care as any other. Actions that individual paramedics might take include completing professional development activities related to the health needs of local minority groups or those that do not regularly come into contact with; this would develop cultural knowledge. Those working in areas with a largely white population might spend a disproportionate time ensuring that they are able to identify and manage conditions such as sickle cell crisis that are more commonly found in Afro-Caribbean communities. Alternatively, if there is a large immigrant population, then paramedics should familiarise themselves with local support services so that they can signpost patients to sources of help.

Direct and indirect discrimination

As well as being negative or positive, discrimination may also be direct or indirect. Direct discrimination is overt, where individuals or groups are specifically targeted for different treatment, e.g. a club that limits its membership by gender. Indirect discrimination can be harder to identify as it describes occasions when a provision, criteria or practice disadvantages a specific group disproportionately, e.g. a uniform requirement that cannot be complied with by certain religious groups. Indirect discrimination may be unintentional but is no less damaging. In certain circumstances, indirect discrimination may be considered legal if it is proportional and is being applied to achieve a legitimate aim. There continues to be some debate around the exclusion of those with medical conditions such as diabetes or epilepsy from driving emergency vehicles. If the employer can show they have made reasonable adjustments, assessed applicants individually and that the requirement is to protect the health and safety of staff and patients, i.e. it is a legitimate aim, and then this would be considered legal. There may also be 'genuine occupational requirements' such as a hostel for women who have suffered domestic abuse advertising for a female paramedic so that clients are less likely to feel vulnerable.

Prejudice

Although not all discrimination is based on prejudice, it lies at the heart of most direct negative discrimination. Prejudices are, as the word suggests, pre-judging someone before identifying their individual merits. This need not always be the obvious categories of race, gender or sexual orientation.

Prejudice has its roots within human psychology, affecting both thoughts and actions. Every minute of every day, there are countless pieces of information bombarding the senses. To try to process every stimulus individually and equally would quickly overwhelm the brain's cognitive abilities. To manage the flow of information, it is categorised based on previous experience or assumptions. Mostly, this is very useful; however, its frequent reliance on assumptions can lead to mistakes. As a very simplistic example, when shown a vehicle with green and yellow checks on the side and blue lights on top for the first time, most people would recognise it as an ambulance. They have seen many ambulances and this has enough in common with those to be placed in the category 'ambulance'. Equally, a red vehicle with blue lights on top might be easily categorised as a 'fire engine'. In using this categorisation approach to ordering information, not only are objects placed into groups but also generalisations are made about the characteristics of these groups. Similarities between objects in the same group are highlighted, e.g. 'all ambulances have first-aid kits' or 'all fire engines have a fire extinguisher'. Differences between the groups are also highlighted, 'ambulances have stretchers but fire engines do not'. These generalisations may or may not be true but make organising the world easier and quicker as they usually hold true. However, there may be occasions when the inference from categorisations may be incorrect, 'ambulances have first-aid kits, this is a fire engine so it will not have a first aid kit'. Just as vehicles may be placed into categories, so people are categorised. The effect of categorising people is further highlighted by the person doing the categorising having to place themselves either in or out of the group. To reinforce our group identity, we highlight the similarities between those in our *in-group* and the differences between ours and other *out-groups* (Walker et al., 2007). The human desire to see oneself in a positive light coupled with this tendency to highlight differences and downplay similarities can lead to bias and potentially prejudicial views.

Discussion point

Think about the occasions when there has been violence between rival groups of sports fans. What are the tangible differences between the groups? If you remove club affiliation, would the two sides be almost indistinguishable from each other? If so, why the violence?

Discussion point

Imagine a paramedic meeting a patient for the first time, how might it affect their approach to that patient if they view them as being members of the same group (perhaps the same ethnic or socio-economic group)? What if they perceive them as being from different groups? How might it affect the (subconscious) value they place on the patient?

As social animals, humans seek to fit into a group and to identify themselves strongly with that group. This served the species well for many centuries where it existed in small groups rarely making contact with anyone from a long distance away. However, with the rise of global travel and communication, there is greater contact with other groups. The increasing size of communities provides us with more categories with which to identify. A further consequence of this is that there are many more people and categories to label as 'other'. This labelling combined with attaching generalisations about the characteristics of those that have been labelled leads to stereotyping (Walker et al., 2007).

In practice, paramedics must be aware of how their fundamental psychology affects the way they look at the world and interact with it. They need to reflect on whether their categorisation of the world is useful and whether it is correct. When meeting a patient who is pale, complaining of breathlessness and chest pain radiating to their left arm categorising them as potentially having a myocardial infarction could be useful as appropriate treatment could be administered more quickly. Attending a patient who has a reduced level of consciousness and is aggressive outside of a pub, the paramedic might categorise them as drunk; this might be less useful, especially if the patient suffers from diabetes. As healthcare professionals, paramedics must be very aware of the prejudices that they carry with them. The way humans think and categorise the world intrinsically lays them open to making unfounded assumptions about people based on their looks and characteristics.

Oppression

Oppression could be considered as a more extreme form of prejudice. In some social work literature, the term anti-oppressive practice is used interchangeably with anti-discriminatory practice. However, there is a differentiation that can be made as oppression refers to the systematic disadvantaging of a group that are discriminated against by another group who are in a more powerful position. If there is prejudice and discrimination between a socially deprived black community and an equally socially deprived Southeast Asian community, it is clearly unacceptable; however, if neither is in a position of power it would not usually constitute oppression. However, prejudice from an established, financially secure community against a recently arrived immigrant population can be oppressive due to the power imbalance between the two groups. The more powerful group has the opportunity to create social structures and cultural norms to reinforce the discrimination of individuals and so institutionalise it. An awareness of how prejudice coupled with a power imbalance can lead to oppressive practices is important to paramedics. Paramedics meet people during very vulnerable periods and as such there is a clear power imbalance that could be open to abuse. When practicing in an anti-discriminatory manner, paramedics should use this imbalance, for example, their better knowledge of the referral options and support available, to counteract any discrimination that the patient encounters.

Equality and diversity

Equality and diversity are central tenets of health strategy. Equality focuses on creating a society where all individuals have the opportunity to reach their full potential without facing unnecessary barriers. Diversity relates to difference, that is recognised and valued for the benefits which it brings. Paramedics look after the full range of patients regardless of socio-economic background, race, ethnicity, gender or sexual orientation and as such an enthusiastic embracing of both equality and diversity is beneficial to their practice.

As health professionals in the 21st century, paramedics should strive to give care to all those individuals on the basis of their clinical need regardless of their background. Caring for such a diverse client base is supported by having a diverse workforce within the profession. Throughout all the public services, there have been problems historically in recruiting from minority groups. Whilst Sir William Macpherson's report (1999) on the inquiry into the death of Stephen Lawrence only identified the Metropolitan Police force as being institutionally racist, it would be naive to think that other public services had an exemplary record then or have not struggled with similar problems since. In the years since the report was published, much progress has been made to ensure that the NHS, ambulance services and the paramedic profession are more representative of the communities that they serve. Anti-discriminatory recruitment practices and positive action have played a role in this; however, many groups are still poorly represented and there is still much work to be done. There is a shortage of research into the ethnic profile of the NHS's workforce and its effects on the care of minority group. This lack of attention could imply that equality and diversity remains a low priority within the NHS as an organisation.

Factors associated with equality

There are many factors that may affect equality as it is experienced by the patients that the paramedics meet in their day to day practice. Some factors are considered so important that there are legislative requirements in the Equality Act 2010 to prevent them. In its guidance to service users on how the Equality Act 2010 applies to healthcare, the Equality and Human Rights Commission (EHRC) identifies seven protected characteristics (EHRC, 2011): disability, gender reassignment, pregnancy and maternity, race, religion or belief, sex, and sexual orientation. It is interesting to note that the EHRC do not identify the protected characteristics of gender reassignment, age, and marriage and civil partnership as applying to healthcare; however, any differences in service that are applied on these grounds would require objective justification. Table 7.1 illustrates the key definitions of protected characteristics adapted from the Equality Act 2010 (part 2, Chapter 1).

Clearly, everyone that paramedics come into contact with in their daily working lives has one or more protected characteristic and as such can be subject to discrimination under the Equality Act 2010. As healthcare professionals, we need to recognise that our patients may face discrimination for a number of reasons. Legally we are required to make reasonable adjustments to cater for patients' protected characteristics, and from an ethical

Table 7.1   Key definitions of protected characteristics

Protected characteristics	Key definitions
Age	Of a particular age group (section 5.1a)
Disability	Physical or mental impairment [*that*] has a substantial and long term adverse effect on [*a person's*] ability to carry out normal day-to-day activities (section 6.1)
Gender reassignment	Proposing to undergo, is undergoing or has undergone a process (or part of a process) for the purpose of reassigning the person's sex by changing physiological or other attributes of sex (section 7.1)
Marriage and civil partnership	Is married or is a civil partner (section 8.1)
Race	Colour, nationality, ethic or national origins. (section 9.1)
Religion means	Any religion including a lack of religion. (section 10.1)
Belief	Any religious or philosophical belief including a lack of belief (section 10.2)
Sex	The characteristics of being a man or a woman (section 11a) and includes discrimination related to breast-feeding, pregnancy and child birth (section 13.6)
Sexual orientation including	Persons of the same sex, opposite sex or either sex (section 12)

Data from Equality Act (2010).

and moral standpoint it is unacceptable to be creating more barriers than they already face.

In addition to those characteristics protected by the Equality Act 2010, we should recognise that there are other factors and characteristics that may lead to our patients experiencing discrimination and there is an ethical obligation even where there is not a legal obligation to challenge any discrimination. Other factors that we should be aware of include discrimination on the grounds of socio-economic status, education, lifestyle choices or appearance. The Health Inequalities report published in 2009 identify poverty, housing and education alongside gender, ethnicity, age, mental health problems and learning disabilities as key areas of health inequality (HSC, 2009). It is especially important that paramedics embrace their legal and ethical obligations to challenge discrimination as the HSC report (2009) suggests marginalised groups are more likely to find themselves at crisis point and calling for paramedic assistance.

Poly-discrimination

When dealing with patients in the real world, it is important to be aware that many experience discrimination from many different directions. A brief look through the list of protected characteristics in the Equality Act 2010 serves to demonstrate that many people have more than one characteristic that may lead them to experiencing discrimination. This effect is referred to as poly-discrimination, and when considering how a patient may be affected by prejudice, paramedics must be aware that it may not be the immediately obvious aspect of their identity that is of concern. In their work on the health status of Gypsies and travellers in England, Parry et al. (2007) took great care to control out socio-economic, gender and home location factors not because these are unimportant but because Gypsies and travellers suffer discrimination due to low income status and because they frequently live in rural or sub-rural settings in addition to inequalities experienced due to their ethnic identity.

Promoting equality

In seeking to work in an anti-discriminatory manner, paramedics should look not only to avoid being discriminatory but also to seek ways to promote equality and reduce the discrimination that some of their patients experience. Whilst it is outside the usual scope of practice of a paramedic to address the wider social barriers that patients may encounter, they have a key role in promoting equality of access to healthcare. This takes the form of providing the best possible care appropriate for that individual and also to provide health promotion advice when coming into contact with those who do not find it easy to access mainstream healthcare.

In any discussion on anti-discriminatory practice it should be remembered that there are potential pitfalls in its realisation. Whilst paramedics must be respectful of cultural differences and be prepared to make appropriate alterations to how they provide treatment they must not be blind to potentially abusive or illegal behaviour. Investigations into tragedies such as the death of Victoria Climbié have highlighted how professionals failed to act on their suspicions of child abuse (Laming, 2003). There is an implication that this was in part due to professionals being either scared of accusations of racism or attributing the carers' actions to cultural differences rather than any sinister motive. When working in a culturally aware manner, paramedics must be mindful that they are trying to provide the same excellent level of care that they do for all their patients in a way that is sympathetic to the patient's culture. Reasonable adjustments should be to facilitate access to healthcare and reduce patients' anxiety. When considering a change in a patient's eventual treatment or destination, the paramedic must be very mindful of why this is being done. For example, if it is suspected a woman has suffered a non-accidental injury, the ultimate aim is to take her to a place of safety and refer her under vulnerable adult guidelines. It should be remembered that there are no cultural, ethnic or socio-economic groups that consider domestic abuse acceptable. Should the paramedic find themselves dealing with someone who claims their culture permits it, that referral is discriminatory or a violation of their beliefs. As a professional, they must be mindful that it remains illegal in the United Kingdom and should act to challenge the evident gender discrimination – probably by involving other services rather than having an argument with the patients or their family. If concerned about accusations of racism they should comfort themselves with the thought that it is preferable to apologise for what later transpires to have been an inappropriate referral than defend their decision not to act in front of the coroner.

Cultural competence/cultural awareness

Paramedics' practice environment brings them into contact with a wide variety of people and with little time to prepare for the interactions. It would be impossible for an individual paramedic to fully understand the culture of every patient that they come into contact with. As such, it is more important that paramedics maintain cultural competence as an approach to their work rather than seeking to fully understand the cultures of every patient that they have the potential to come into contact with. When working in an area where a particular cultural group make up a significant part of the population, it may be useful to seek out information about that group's cultural norms. It is important to remember the tendency to generalise and assume similarity within a group. There is frequently more difference within a group than there is between groups and care should still be taken not to make too many assumptions. Despite the preceding assertion, there is one culture that a paramedic must have a detailed and conscious awareness of and that is their own. The first step towards practising in a culturally aware manner is to be aware of one's own assumptions, beliefs and values. This self-awareness is not sufficient to achieve an anti-discriminatory way of practising but is a first step. There is a risk that having identified their own cultural norms, the paramedic may decide that whilst other cultural identities may exist theirs is the best and consequently others are less desirable or inferior. The aim of a culturally competent paramedic should be an awareness of their own values and the potential impact they may have on interactions with patients. They should be constantly looking for and questioning assumptions that may be misinterpreted, cause misunderstandings or offence.

At first, individual patient-centred cultural awareness may appear difficult to achieve, however, it is in reality an extension of what the paramedic does during any patient contact in looking for information, signs and symptoms and trying to link them together to come to a treatment plan. It would be a very naive paramedic who assumed that chest pain is only very cardiac in origin, or that Entonox is the only way in which to treat pain; as such, it is a very naive paramedic that assumes that not making eye contact is always a sign of insincerity or that everyone of Asian appearance is a Muslim.

Education

Some individuals will enter the paramedic profession with well-established cultural competence; however, many will not and all will benefit from ensuring that they can practise in a culturally competent and non-discriminatory manner. It is outside the scope of this text to provide a comprehensive course in developing cultural competence. As discussed earlier, there is a legal requirement on organisations providing public healthcare, whether they are NHS or independent providers that they encourage anti-discriminatory practice and most paramedics will have been involved in some form of equality and diversity training during their employment. The purpose of the final part of this chapter is to discuss some of the concepts underlying education in cultural competence and to promote what Campinha-Bacote (2002) refers to as *cultural desire*, paramedics who *want* to be culturally competent rather than feeling they *have* to as part of their role.

Care should be taken when developing cultural competence to avoid a reductionist or purely fact-based approach. Identifying key facts about a commonly encountered group has its place. However, there is a risk of ethnic stereo-typing and as such any 'facts' must be tempered with an awareness of intragroup variability and that to have a comprehensive

factual knowledge of all groups that a clinician may encounter is impractical (American Institutes for Research, 2002). Regarding intragroup variability it is worth reiterating 'There is more variation within ethnic groups
than across ethnic groups' (Campinha-Bacote, 2002) and as such a person-
centred approach is most effective when planning culturally sensitive care
in paramedic practice just as it is in wider health and social care settings.
Much of the literature relating to the development of cultural competency
has arisen from the United States. Whilst the healthcare system is very different from that of the United Kingdom, the aim is transferable across the
Atlantic. That is, addressing the needs of marginalised groups in accessing
care in a system that has grown up based on the needs, and research data,
from a largely white middle-class population (Salmond, 1999).

It has already been mentioned that the first step toward anti-
discriminatory practice and cultural competence is to be *culturally aware* of
one's own beliefs. Every paramedic is a member of a cultural group (in fact,
several) and the process of cultural competency begins with an honest appraisal of their own biases, prejudices and assumptions (Campinha-Bacote,
2002) to avoid the trap of imposing their own norms on other cultures. That
the religious and ethnic identity of a clinician can affect their decision making has been demonstrated by Seale (2010). Once aware of their own beliefs,
paramedics require *cultural knowledge* about ethnic groups, the previous
caution against a reductionist approach notwithstanding. Lavizzo-Mourey
and Mackenzie (1996) suggest that this knowledge can be sub-divided into
beliefs and values, disease incidence and treatment efficacy. Examples of
where this may be important are an acceptance of the differences between
cultural groups of the importance of home and family. Despite the medical view of a patient's chronic condition indicating transfer to hospital
for aggressive treatment if that patient's cultural identity places a higher
value on remaining in the care of the family at home at the time of death,
it may be most appropriate to arrange palliative care at home via community services. It has also been previously mentioned that certain conditions
have different rates of incidence between ethnic groups, e.g. cardiovascular
disease and diabetes are more prevalent in men of Southeast Asian origin
(Simmons et al., 1991; Knight et al., 1992; Wild and McKeique, 1997) and
the efficacy of certain treatments varies. Gibbs et al. (1999a) highlighted the
reduced efficacy of beta-blockers and ACE inhibitors in patients of African
origin and their greater risk of suffering angioedema following ACE in-
hibitor treatment (Gibbs et al., 1999b). This is now supported by the National Institute for Health and Clinical Excellence (NICE) (2011) and British
Hypertension Society guidelines. However, considering the limited formulary available to paramedics, treatment efficacy has a lesser impact on their
decision making. Since it is not possible for the paramedic to have complete cultural knowledge of every potential group they might encounter,
Campinha-Bacote (2002) identifies the next step as developing *cultural skill*.
This is being able to gather relevant cultural information that may affect an

individual's condition, and also being able to tailor physical assessments to be culturally appropriate. For the inexperienced paramedic trying to gather cultural information may just mean being prepared to ask questions. It is unlikely that a patient will be offended by a question regarding their cultural beliefs or practices; and if they are, then they are likely to be more offended by clumsy attempts to make allowances for beliefs they do not hold. Paramedics must be able to conduct a physical assessment appropriate to a patient's ethnic background; this may require consideration of cultural practices or the effect of a patient's body structure or skin pigmentation to physiological norms. For example, cyanosis in an Afro-Caribbean patient may be more difficult to detect than in those of Caucasian origin. As with any skill cultural competency requires practice, it requires *cultural encounters*. Personal cultural awareness and textbook cultural knowledge need to be moderated by repeated exposure to different cultural groups, ideally in and out of the clinical setting. A medical emergency is not the best time to be gaining cultural knowledge or honing cultural skills. Time spent with diverse groups outside of the clinical environment will be of great use when circumstances are more urgent. The more exposure the clinician has to cultural groups, the better their cultural skills will be, and less prone to stereotyping. As stated at the beginning of this section, the strongest impetus to the process of developing cultural competency is cultural desire. Possessing a real wish to meet the needs of every patient taking account of their individual needs, be these culturally or clinically based, should be the ambition of every paramedic.

Summary

This chapter has introduced the concepts of anti-discriminatory practice and cultural competency. The cognitive basis of discrimination has been explored, where it may be useful as an aid to rapid decision making and where it can evolve into prejudice and possibly oppression. Discrimination and its avoidance has been considered such an important issue for a country as diverse as the United Kingdom that it has been the focus of a number of laws over the past decades culminating most recently in the Equality Act 2010. It is hoped that the reader will understand the reasons for this and how they relate to their practice as a paramedic. As awareness of its importance is only a first step along the path to develop the skills required for cultural competence. Different readers will be at different points along that path, however, all will be aiming to reach a position where they can interact comfortably with any patient they encounter. To do so requires self-awareness, knowledge, skills and a willingness to engage and use them.

It is hoped that no one enters into the paramedic profession seeking to shore up and encourage discrimination against any group. Paramedics care deeply about their patients and the care they provide. To meet a person in distress, needing help, who has previously felt excluded by mainstream society and then to ensure they are made to feel comfortable, valued and cared for in a personalised way, meeting their needs both clinical and cultural is the greatest skills that a paramedic can possess and will give the greatest job satisfaction. To do so is not easy and requires time and effort to achieve. The development of cultural desire not only enhances a paramedic's practice but also their life and the lives of those around them.

Critical thinking

ALEXEJ'S FOOT

Jamie is solo responding and has been called to a building site where the foreman is concerned because one of his workers is unable to walk due to a foot injury. Sat in the site office is Alexej who has an open sore on the ball of his foot. Alexej has difficulty explaining what has happened, he apologises that his English is not very good. The site foreman explains that Alexej has recently moved to the United Kingdom to work in the building trade and although he usually has good English, the worry about his foot means that he is struggling today.

Jamie is concerned that the wound looks infected and may have happened sometime ago. It is challenging to get any more information from Alexej, so an ambulance is requested to transport him to the nearest accident and emergency (A&E) department where hopefully they can sort out his foot. Alexej looks worried about having to go to the hospital and Jamie wonders whether this may be due to his immigration status.

When the ambulance arrives, the paramedic on board, Sam, takes the handover from Jamie and has a look at Alexej's foot. Sam is also concerned that the injury does not look recent and Alexej's apparent reluctance to attend hospital. Drawing on previous experience, Sam starts to ask Alexej some more detailed questions as there is a suspicion that the injury may be secondary to an underlying condition.

On further questioning and keeping the language simple, Sam discovers that Alexej has type 1 diabetes. He registered with a local GP as soon as he arrived in the country to arrange the prescription for his insulin; however, that is on repeat and he does not have the time to see the GP during surgery hours as he is working to send money home to his family. Alexej is living with five other men so that they can afford the rent on the small flat they share. On further questioning, Sam discovers that Alexej is concerned that an ambulance journey to A&E will be very expensive and he will not be able to afford the bill. Sam assures him that he will not be charged for the journey or any treatment. Referral through the specialist diabetic nurse is discussed as Sam knows that an outreach clinic for those who can only attend outside normal office hours has recently been set up. Alexej is grateful for the information and

Sam says there should be information leaflets available at the hospital translated into his first language.

- What were Jamie's initial assumptions about Alexej? How did Jamie go about challenging or confirming these assumptions?
- How did Jamie and Sam's approaches differ?
- What potential areas of discrimination does Alexej face? Which has acted as the greatest barrier to accessing healthcare in this case?
- What services were identified to overcome these barriers?
- Think about when you first read through this case study, did you assign a gender to Jamie and Sam? If so, why do you think you chose that gender, albeit subconsciously?
- Did you ascribe any other racial or socio-economic characteristics to either paramedic? Did either of them resemble you and if so was it with Sam or Jamie that you identified the closest?

References

American Institutes for Research (2002) *Teaching Cultural Competence in Healthcare: review of current concepts, policies and practices*. Report prepared for the Office of Minority Health. Washington DC.

Beauchamp, T.L. & Childress, J.F. (1977) *Principles of Biomedical Ethics*. Oxford University Press, New York.

Beauchamp, T.L. & Childress, J.F. (2001) *Principles of Biomedical Ethics*. 6th edn. Oxford University Press, New York.

Campinha-Bacote, J. (2002) The process of cultural competency in the delivery of healthcare services: A model of care. *Journal of Transcultural Nursing*, **13**(3), 181–184.

Equality and Human Rights Commission (2011) *Your Rights to Equality from Healthcare and Social Care Services: Equality Act 2010 Guidance of your rights. Volume 5 of 9*. EHRC, London.

Gibbs, C.R., Lip, G.Y.H. & Beevers, D.G. (1999a) The management of hypertensive disease in black patients. *QJM*, **92**(8), 481.

Gibbs, C.R., Lip, G.Y.H. & Beevers, D.G. (1999b) Angioedema due to ACE inhibitors: increased risk in patients of African origin. *British Journal of Clinical Pharmacology*, **48**(6), 861–865.

Health & Care Professions Council (2012) *Standards of Proficiency: Paramedics*. HCPC, London.

Health Select Committee (2009) Health Inequalities: The role of the NHS in tackling health inequalities. *Health Select Committee Publications* London: Parliament. Available at http://www.publications.parliament.uk/pa/cm200809/cmselect/cmhealth/286/28609.htm (accessed 29th March 2012)

Iserson, K.V., Sanders, A.B., & Mathieu, D. (1995) *Ethics in Emergency Medicine*, 2nd edn. Galen Press, Tucson.

Knight, T.M., Smith, Z., Whittles, A., et al. (1992) Insulin resistance, diabetes, and risk markers for ischemic heart disease in Asian men and non-Asian in Bradford. *British Heart Journal*, **67**(5), 343–350.

Laming (2003) *The Victoria Climbié Inquiry: Report.* Stationery Office, London.

Lavizzo-Mourey, R. & Mackenzie, E.R. (1996). Cultural competence: Essential measurements of quality for managed care organizations. *Annals of Internal Medicine.* **124**(10), 919–921.

Macpherson, W. (1999) *The Stephen Lawrence Inquiry.* Stationery Office, London.

NHS Employers (2005) Positive Action in the NHS. NHS Employers Briefing Issue. 10, October 2005. Available at http://www.nhsemployers.org/Aboutus/Publications/Documents/postive_action_briefing_10_151005.pdf (accessed 29th March 2012)

National Institute for Health and Clinical Excellence (2011) *NICE Clinical Guideline 127 Hypertension: Clinical Management of Primary Hypertension in Adults.* NICE, London.

Parry, G., van Cleemput, P., Peters, J., et al. (2007) Health Status of Gypsies and travellers in England. *Journal of Epidemiology and Community Health.* **61**(3), 198–204.

Quality Assurance Agency (2004) *Benchmark Statement: Health Care Programmes - Paramedic Science.* QAA, London.

Salmond, S.W. (1999) Managed care: Pitfalls for cultural bias. *Journal of Transcultural Nursing.* **10**(4), 295–296.

Scullion, P. (2000) Anti-discriminatory practice: Do health professionals need it? *British Journal of Therapy and Rehabilitation.* **7**(4), 157.

Seale, C. (2010) The role of doctors' religious faith and ethnicity in taking ethically controversial decisions during end-of-life care. *Journal of Medical Ethics.* **36**(11), 677–682.

Simmons, D., Williams, D.R. & Powell, M.J. (1991) The Coventry Diabetes Study: prevalence of diabetes and impaired glucose tolerance in Europids and Asians. *The Quarterly Journal of Medicine.* **81**(296), 1021–1030.

Thompson, N. (2005) *Anti-Discriminatory Practice,* 4th edn. Palgrave Macmillan, Basingstoke.

Walker, J., Payne, S., Smith, P. & Jarrett, N. (2007) *Psychology for Nurses and the Caring Professions.* McGraw Hill, Maidenhead.

Wild, S. & Mckeique, P. (1997) Cross sectional analysis of mortality by country of birth in England and Wales, 1970-92. *British Medical Journal.* **314**(7082), 705–710.

Table of Statutes

Disability Discrimination Act 2005
Equal Pay Act 1970
Equality Act 2010
Mental Capacity Act 2005
Race Relations (amendment) Act 2000
Sex Discrimination Act 1975

8 Medicines Management

Lorna McInulty

School of Health, University of Central Lancashire, Preston, UK

Introduction to medicines management

Medicines management and drug therapy are integral parts of clinical practice for most healthcare professionals working in emergency and urgent care. In clinical practice, the terms 'medicine' and 'drug' are often used synonymously but, in fact, have slightly different meanings and implications. Whereas a 'drug' may be defined as a chemical or substance, not necessarily for medical purposes, that alters the way the mind or body works, a 'medicine' is used strictly for the purpose of diagnosing, treating or preventing disease. This chapter will therefore refer largely to 'medicines'.

The chapter will be of relevance to paramedics, generic emergency nurses, emergency nurse practitioners (ENPs) and those working in the role of emergency care practitioner (ECP). This latter role is often seen as a form of career progression for paramedics and nurses but may also be undertaken by other suitably qualified and experienced healthcare professionals, such as physiotherapists. The difference between an ENP and an ECP is that the ENP is a registered nurse working mainly in emergency departments (EDs) and walk-in centres, who can assess, treat and discharge a range of patients, presenting with minor injuries or illness, usually under strict protocol, but without reference to a doctor. An ECP, however, may derive from a number of different professions – often, nursing and physiotherapy but more commonly paramedic practice. The work of the ECP is not confined to the ED or walk-in centre but may include mobile healthcare and care in the patient's own home. The ECP has been described as 'occupying the space between the general practitioner (GP), the nurse and the paramedic' (Doy and Turner, 2004).

Experience has shown that as each of the above professions has developed, and continues to do so, so too has the range of skills and treatments involving the use of medicines. Nurses working in emergency care have

Professional Practice in Paramedic, Emergency and Urgent Care, First Edition. Edited by Val Nixon.
© 2013 John Wiley & Sons, Ltd. Published 2013 by John Wiley & Sons, Ltd.

seen their roles grow and develop very rapidly since the publication of the document, 'Reforming Emergency Care' (Department of Health (DH), 2001). This document was the impetus for the nationwide establishment of roles such as ENP and also for increasing the clinical responsibilities of the more generic emergency nurse, for example the provision of medicines to patients at triage, without the need to first refer them to a doctor. A natural progression from looking at ways of improving care in the ED was to consider the role and function of the ambulance service. As a result of on-going review of the ambulance service (DH, 2005; Association of Ambulance Chief Executives, 2011), it is the paramedic profession that is currently developing at the most rapid pace, with an increasing range of medicines being made available for paramedic use, in both traditional and non-traditional ambulance settings.

The necessary underpinning knowledge required for safe clinical practice in medicines management is therefore paramount and includes knowledge of the law as it relates to medicines; an understanding of the potential ethical issues that may result in the course of medicine administration; professional issues around medicines management, as well as the clinical knowledge required around medicines; their indications; their actions and interactions. The importance of all these issues cannot be over-emphasised; however, this chapter will mainly explore the legal and professional knowledge that the practitioner should possess for safe and competent practice. Topics that will be covered include the Medicines Act of 1968, the Misuse of Drugs Act (1971), the legal classifications of drugs, the role of prescription only exemptions in clinical practice and the use of Patient Group Directions (PGDs). Progress regarding non-medical prescribing will be described and the importance and relevance of continuing professional development will be demonstrated in relation to all of these aspects of safe medicines management.

Introduction to the Medicines Act

The legitimate manufacture, sale and supply of drugs are all tightly controlled by legislation deriving from the Medicines Act of 1968. The Act is also concerned with the storage and use of all medicinal products. Responsibility for enforcing and monitoring the Act lies with the Medicines and Healthcare Products Regulatory Agency (MHRA) – an executive agency of the Department of Health, which was formed in 2003 following the merger of the Medicines Control Agency, previously established as a result of the Medicines Act, and the Medical Devices Agency. Consequently, as well as regulating medicine safety, the MHRA also has a role in relation to the safety and regulation of all medical devices. By applying monitoring and tight controls to medicines management, both the public and the professions can be reassured that any medications they may respectively take or administer have been developed, stored and supplied in a quality-assured manner that implies clinical safety.

The Medicines Act (1968) clearly delineates exactly who can prescribe, supply or administer drugs and is therefore of great significance to all healthcare professionals. Because of the changing nature of society and the concurrent development of a number of different healthcare professions, the original Act has been revised a number of times in order to remain relevant.

Prescribing, supplying and administering drugs

To understand the Act in detail, it is important that practitioners have a clear understanding of the terms used within it such as 'prescribe', 'supply' and 'administer'. To 'prescribe' is to authorise in writing the supply of a medicine for a named patient (DH, 1999). To be deemed able to prescribe, a function that was previously only in the domain of doctors and dentists, requires that non-medical registered practitioners undergo a validated course of further study that leads specifically to a pertinent qualification. 'Supply' describes the provision of a medicine to a patient (or carer) for administration, and to 'administer' refers to the physical act of giving a medication to a patient, e.g. orally or by injection (DH, 1999).

Categorisation of drugs

The Medicines Act (1968) determines three different categories into which all drugs fall. These are known as:

- Prescription only medicines (POM)
- Pharmacy medicines (P)
- General Sales List medicines (GSL)

GSL medicines include common remedies such as Paracetamol, Ibuprofen, Aspirin and Clotrimazole which can be purchased by members of the public in shops as well as in pharmacies, and indeed from any lockable business premises. Pharmacy medicines do not require a prescription but may only be supplied under the supervision of a pharmacist. The pharmacist's responsibility is to ensure that the drug is appropriate for the purpose for which the person intends to use it and to check that it is unlikely to have any adverse effects, based on the person's general health or on any potential interactions with other medication that the person may be taking. In terms of the ambulance service, ambulance Trusts can legally obtain pharmacy medicines into their stock and there are no legal restrictions on who can administer them. Examples of pharmacy medicines include Chloramphenicol and Omeprazole, though it is important to recognise that not all strengths of the same medicine may have the same classification. For example, only 10 mg Omeprazole may be supplied under pharmacy conditions (Royal Pharmaceutical Society, 2004), whereas greater strengths of this medication still require a prescription. Collectively, pharmacy and GSL medicines are often referred to as 'over-the-counter' (OTC) medications although this is not a formal and legal classification. Registered nurses, paramedics and ambulance technicians can all administer GSLs.

POMs require a prescription from a suitably qualified healthcare practitioner. Formerly, this meant that only a dentist, doctor or GP could prescribe medicines but with the development of healthcare, many other professionals are now recognised as prescribers, following a suitably approved programme of education. Prescribing can be either independent or supplementary. Independent prescribing means that the professional possesses the skills to fully assess a patient and prescribe for them as part of their care (Lawson and Hennefer, 2010). Supplementary means that the professional can prescribe any medicine, including controlled drugs, for any condition within their scope of competence, but only under a clinical management plan agreed with both an independent prescriber and the patient concerned (Courtenay and Griffiths, 2007).

Non-medical prescribing

Currently, prescribing extends to nurses, pharmacists, physiotherapists and optometrists, amongst others, with the caveat that all individual professionals prescribe within their own scope of practice. Once originated by a prescriber, those practitioners supplying and administering the medication must follow the directions on the prescription precisely. In some circumstances, a prescription may be given verbally but must be followed by a written prescription within 24 hours (Davies, 2011). Recent consultations have taken place with regard to paramedic prescribing (DH, 2010a) but as yet, no firm edict has emerged that has allowed the profession to progress in this respect.

The arguments in favour of paramedic prescribing are described in the initial engagement document released by the Department of Health (DH, 2010a) prior to the undertaking of a formal consultation on the subject. This stakeholder engagement followed the influential paper, 'Taking Healthcare to the Patient' (DH, 2005) in which the concept of paramedic prescribing was first actively explored. In the stakeholder engagement, paramedics described many and varied situations in which a prescribing qualification could have prevented a patient from calling out a GP; being referred on to another practitioner or having to attend the ED, e.g. for a lost inhaler. Paramedic prescribing would also sit very comfortably within the ethos of a patient-centred health service, supporting the accessibility of medicines to the public. However, arguments against paramedic prescribing include the notion that the most intensive training of the paramedic has been concentrated on the sickest of patients whilst the reality is that 90% of the paramedic workload is more mundane and often of a primary care nature (DH, 2005). Therefore, for a paramedic to be able to prescribe appropriately may require significant further education and development.

The current educational background of a paramedic might give cause for concern as until the relatively recent move to higher education, a paramedic might have qualified after as little as 6 weeks of very practically orientated in-service training which did not address the development of critical thinking skills. As paramedics remain one of the few healthcare professionals who can register to a professional body without a degree-level education, they are currently not in harmony with modern healthcare developments and may be disadvantaged as a result. Until the inception of the Health Care Professions (now the Health and Care Professions Council (HCPC)), the notion of on-going professional development for paramedics was not a professional requirement but more a personal choice. Furthermore, some studies have identified a lack of basic numeracy skills amongst paramedics (Eastwood et al., 2009) and student paramedics (Eastwood et al., 2011a) which could further disarm the paramedic, particularly in a multi-professional situation such as is advocated for non-medical prescribing courses. However, it is interesting to note that similar numeracy problems have been highlighted amongst nursing and medical practitioners too (McMullan et al., 2010; McQueen et al., 2010; Axe, 2011; Eastwood et al., 2011b).

Proposals surrounding eligibility for paramedic prescribing are quite rightly stringent and require that the paramedic be able to function at a quite high level of professional expertise, equating to level 7 competencies on the 'Skills for Health Careers Framework' (www.skillsforhealth.org.uk). Enhanced assessment skills, differential diagnosis and referral rights would also be necessary. Although different 'levels' or options for prescribing exist (see Box 8.1) and would have to be agreed upon, it remains that

---

Box 8.1   Options for paramedic prescribing

- No change, continuing to use Patient Group Directions (PGDs) and Exemptions for supply and/or administration of medicines
- Supplementary prescribing
- Prescribing for specified conditions from a specified formulary of medicines
- Prescribing for any condition from a specified formulary
- Prescribing for specific medical conditions from a full formulary (within competence)
- Prescribing for any condition from a full formulary (within competence)

Data from DH (2010a).

appropriate educational programmes would have to be undertaken in order to qualify as a prescriber, and in reality, only a small percentage of paramedics might currently be considered educationally and professionally prepared to take on such an endeavour.

More positively, non-medical prescribing is now well established and has demonstrated safe outcomes and patient satisfaction (Courtenay and Griffiths, 2007). Therefore, the experience of other professional groups can be of value in helping to progress paramedic prescribing, particularly the experience of nursing which endured,

'a long and protracted introduction to nurse prescribing over a period of 15 years [which] culminated in … an extremely limited formulary at least in its infancy'. (Tinson, 2007, p. 51)

POMs exemptions

With regard to POMs, there are important exemptions that affect all paramedics registered with the HCPC. These exemptions originate from an update to the Medicines Act (1968) and allow the paramedic to administer certain parenteral drugs without prescription (see Box 8.2), for the immediate and necessary treatment of sick or injured persons (Prescription Only Medicine (Human Use) Order (1997).

Legally, such parenteral drugs can only be administered by a registered professional. However, with regard to administration of such drugs by student paramedics, The College of Paramedics, the professional body for paramedic practice, has recently lobbied the MHRA in a bid to change the legislation surrounding this aspect of care and expects that the MHRA will be consulting with the DH imminently to agree the actions required (Collen, 2012). The College's stance follows a precedent set by the Royal College of Midwives who argued that it was unreasonable and indeed unsafe to expect a newly registered practitioner to administer a parenteral drug having never had the opportunity of doing so whilst a student (College of Paramedics, 2011a). The College of Paramedics seeks to redress this to enable students in their final year to practice this skill whilst still under the supervision of a qualified mentor, 'within a robust governance and assurance framework' (College of Paramedics, 2011b). This is on the basis, that although newly qualified paramedics should be provided with a suitable period of preceptorship, this is not guaranteed and consequently, the first time they perform the administration of a parenteral medicine, it could quite feasibly be entirely unsupervised.

Further to the POM exemptions, a second list of parenteral drugs exists that can be administered by 'anybody' in a life-saving emergency (see Box 8.3). The overarching law around medicines states that no one can

> **Box 8.2   POM exemptions for registered paramedics**
>
> - Diazepam 5 mg per ml emulsion for injection
> - Succinylated modified fluid gelatin 4% intravenous infusion
> - POMs containing one or more of the following substances but no other active ingredient:
>   - Adrenaline acid tartrate
>   - Amiodarone
>   - Anhydrous glucose
>   - Benzylpenicillin
>   - Bretylium tosylate
>   - Compound sodium lactate intravenous infusion (Hartmann's solution)
>   - Ergometrine maleate
>   - Furosemide
>   - Glucose
>   - Heparin sodium (NB: administration is only allowed for the purpose of cannula flushing)
>   - Lidocaine hydrochloride
>   - Metoclopramide
>   - Morphine sulphate
>   - Nalbuphine hydrochloride
>   - Naloxone hydrochloride
>   - Polygeline
>   - Reteplase
>   - Sodium bicarbonate
>   - Sodium chloride
>   - Streptokinase
>   - Syntometrine
>   - Tenecteplase
>
> Data from MHRA (2005).

administer a parenteral medicine to anyone except himself unless he is an appropriate practitioner or acting in accordance with the directions of an appropriate practitioner. The medicines on this list, however, are exempt from this restriction when administered for the purpose of saving a life in an emergency. The list differs from the POM exemptions described previously and includes, for example Atropine and Hydrocortisone which are sometimes administered by paramedics. Despite the terminology used to describe this list of drugs, the healthcare professional does not have carte blanche to administer them, as element of training would still be necessary to support safe practice.

> **Box 8.3   Drugs that can be administered in a life-threatening emergency**
>
> - Adrenaline injection 1 in 1000 (1 mg in 1 ml)
> - Atropine sulphate injection
> - Atropine sulphate and obidoxime chloride injection
> - Atropine sulphate and pralidoxime chloride injection
> - Atropine sulphate, pralidoxime mesilate and avizafone injection
> - Chlorphenamine injection
> - Dicobalt edetate injection
> - Glucagon injection
> - Glucose injection 50%
> - Hydrocortisone injection
> - Naloxone hydrochloride
> - Pralidoxime chloride injection
> - Pralidoxime mesilate injection
> - Promethazine hydrochloride injection
> - Snake venom antiserum
> - Sodium nitrite injection
> - Sodium thiosulphate injection
> - Sterile pralidoxime
>
> Data from MHRA (2010).

Amendments to the medicines act

As stated previously, amendments are sometimes made to The Medicines Act in order to progress clinical practice. An example of this occurred in relation to the Prescription Only Medicines (Human Use) Order of 1977, in early 2003/2004, when a number of more modern thrombolytic agents (Tenecteplase and Reteplase) were proposed for paramedic use, in preference to the then first-line drug Streptokinase which was administered to patients with acute myocardial infarction. In order to achieve this, a consultation letter was distributed by the Medicines and Healthcare Products Regulatory Agency to 'all interested organisations' outlining the proposals (MHRA, 2003). 'Interested organisations' might include the Joint Royal Colleges Ambulance Liaison Committee (JRCALC); all ambulance Trusts; other healthcare professionals from relevant specialities and relevant professional bodies such as the HCPC, the General Medical Council, the Royal Colleges and the Royal Pharmaceutical Society. Individual practitioners can also usually respond to such proposals.

In this particular example, the proposals centred around the recognition that the drug Streptokinase was perhaps not best suited to the pre-hospital environment because of the requirement for very precisely controlled infusion, as well as the incidence of allergic reactions to it, including anaphylaxis. The drugs Tenecteplase and Reteplase were considered safer in respect to allergenicity and additionally had the advantage of bolus administration.

When such a consultation takes place, a period of time is allowed for all interested parties to respond and it is usual to make all comments publicly available unless a respondent specifically indicates to the contrary. Following this, all responses are collated and examined and after due consideration of the risks and benefits, a recommendation is made and conveyed to government ministers. A decision is then taken as to whether or not the proposal can become law, which in this case it did.

Clearly, not all drugs advocated for use by paramedics are classified as POM exemptions or as parenteral medicines that can be administered by anybody for the purpose of saving a life in an emergency. Analgesics and antipyretics, such as Paracetamol, do not fall into this category but are regularly administered by paramedics. It is also important to recognise that POM exemptions do not apply to nurses and physiotherapists yet the modernisation of emergency care, along with the development of urgent care centres and walk-in centres, does demand that all of these healthcare professionals provide a wider range of medicines to patients than was previously the case. In these situations, medicines are often administered under what is known as a PGD.

Discussion point

A community matron regularly attends a known and brittle asthmatic patient who is house bound. On one particular visit, the patient presents with an acute exacerbation of asthma, diagnosed through the matron's thorough history taking, clinical examination and evaluation of the clinical findings, based on best evidence produced by the British Thoracic Society. The patient has an agreed management plan, developed in collaboration with the both the patient and the patient's GP. On this basis, the matron decides to prescribe a course of oral steroids. What type of prescribing is described in this scenario? Do you think it is relevant to your own present role?

Patient group directions

Patient Group Directions (PGDs) (formerly known as Patient Group Directives) allow the healthcare professional to administer, *directly* to the patient, other medications that are neither POM exemptions nor of a life-saving nature, but which may enhance patient care and comfort. PGDs are therefore more likely to be used by paramedics working in non-traditional roles, such as the Emergency Care Practitioner, and are commonly used by emergency nurses. PGDs were first instituted in the year 2000 and constitute a legal framework which allows certain registered healthcare professionals to supply and administer medicines to non-specified individual patients, without the patient seeing a prescriber, on the proviso that the patient fits the criteria laid out in the PGD (National Prescribing Centre (NPC), 2009). The legal definition of a PGD is:

> 'A written instruction for the sale, supply and/or administration of named medicines in an identified clinical situation. It applies to groups of patients who may not be individually identified before presenting for treatment'. (NPC, 2009, p. 11)

This latter point highlights the main difference between a PGD and a prescription. A prescription which can be referred to as a Patient Specific Direction (PSD) is used once a patient has been assessed by a prescriber and has a written instruction to instruct a qualified healthcare professional to supply or administer a medicine to that *named individual* (NPS, 2009). PGDs are not intended for long term use but rather as a short term measure in situations where medicine use is largely predictable but not necessarily individualised. Therefore, their use is ideal for non-medical practitioners working in urgent care centres, walk-in centres and EDs. As already identified, the use of PGDs is very different from prescribing and should not be described as such. Those who utilise PGDs must be suitably qualified and trained in their application (NPC, 2009) and additionally, must be individually named. A record of the names and signatures of the designated individuals is usually kept by a relevant and appropriately nominated person within the employing organisation.

Legally, the PGD itself must be reviewed every 2 years, otherwise it becomes invalid. However, if clinical practice changes in the interim period, the PGD should be similarly amended at that point. All records of signatories and all PGDs should be reviewed regularly to ensure good practice. Authorised employees who use PGDs should check that in the event of a mistake or allegation of clinical negligence, they are protected by their Trust's vicarious liability. It is also vitally important that they secure professional indemnity insurance, as advocated for those who advance their roles into areas that place them at higher risk of clinical negligence allegations through acts or omissions in practice (Broadhead, 2011). A healthcare professional who utilises a PGD that is not currently in date would be acting outside the law and would be liable and accountable, legally and professionally, for his or her actions.

At around the same time that PGDs were legalised, the DH developed templates and guidelines for their production and subsequent clinical use.

PGDs must be developed in a multidisciplinary manner and must at least involve a pharmacist, a doctor and a representative of the professional group for whom the PGD is intended (Royal College of Nursing, 2004). Once developed, the PGD must be formally approved by a designated person in the organisation, often a clinical governance lead. This person, along with the pharmacist and doctor involved, must be signatories to the PGD.

Legislation requires that PGDs contain the following information:

- The name of the body to which the direction applies
- The date the direction comes into force and the date it expires
- A description of the medicine(s) to which the direction applies
- The clinical conditions covered by the direction
- A description of those patients excluded from treatment under the direction
- A description of the circumstances under which further advice should be sought from a doctor (or dentist, as appropriate) and arrangements for referral made
- Appropriate dosage and maximum total dosage, quantity, pharmaceutical form and strength, route and frequency of administration, and minimum or maximum period over which the medicine should be administered
- Relevant warnings, including potential adverse reactions
- Details of any follow-up action and the circumstances
- A statement of the records to be kept for audit purposes

(NPC, 2009)

In the culture of sharing good practice, DH-approved templates and many examples of PGDs are available to healthcare professionals on the National Electronic Library for Health PGD website (www.nelm.nhs.uk). These can either be adopted exactly as presented or adapted by individual organisations to meet their own requirements. Because there is sometimes confusion around PGDs and other methods of providing drugs and medication, a useful flow chart is also available on the website to help organisations make the right decision.

Training for PGDs

Although there are national templates, there is no national training programme for PGDs and the responsibility for this lies within each individual organisation. There is, however, a competency framework available from the NPC (NPC, 2009) which can be used by organisations in an attempt to ensure practitioners are properly prepared to supply and administer drugs under PGD. Within the framework, there are nine competencies covering three domains. The domains are

1. the consultation
2. effective supply and administration using a PGD
3. PGDs in context.

The consultation element requires the practitioner to have the requisite clinical and pharmaceutical knowledge, as well as the ability to communicate effectively with patients, in order to establish management options. The second domain relates to safe use of the PGD, professional standards and practice development. The third domain encompasses PGD information, NHS information, and both the team and the individual in context. For all domains, the competency statements are clearly defined. The framework is intended for multidisciplinary use and can be applied in any clinical setting. Additionally, it is recommended for use as an audit tool to benchmark existing training and development programmes, to ensure that all the required PGD competencies are being addressed.

Grey areas in medicines management

Despite the many guidance documents for PGDs, grey areas can still occur in practice when medicines which are to be administered do not belong to either the POM exemption list or the list of medicines that can be given by anyone in an emergency for the purpose of saving a life. As an example of one potentially confusing situation, a PGD is not in fact legally necessary to administer a GSL medicine. Nevertheless, nurses frequently utilise a PGD in these circumstances, e.g. to administer Paracetamol. This is because the Nursing and Midwifery Council (NMC) (2010) dictates that nurses can only administer medicines under the following conditions:

- Patient group directions
- Patient-specific directions
- Patient medicines administration chart
- Medicines Act exemption (where it applies to nurses)
- Standing order
- Home remedy protocol
- Prescription forms

This explains why EDs have PGDs for GSL medicines. However, there should be no confusion over the fact that a PGD is necessary to supply pharmacy medicines, unless the supply is being made at a registered pharmacy by or under the supervision of a pharmacist.

Non-nursing organisations, which are not subject to the NMC's requirements, may opt to use a simple protocol for GSL medicines to guide their practitioners. For example, the North West Ambulance Service (NWAS), in order to minimise clinical error, opts to use a 'Drug Administration Protocol Reference Guide' (NWAS, 2009) for both paramedics and technicians, in which all drugs, dosages, indications and contraindications are presented in a similar manner regardless of whether they are POM or GSL. The guide states exactly who can administer each drug, whether paramedic or technician. This ensures appropriate clinical governance is in place.

When compared to the higher numbers of PGDs used in EDs, urgent care and walk-in centres, most of the drugs used in paramedic practice are either POM exemption or GSL. Again, using the NWAS as an example, this organisation currently includes only a very small number of PGDs in its formulary, one example being Enoxaparin (NWAS, 2009), as this does not fall into either POM or GSL categories.

Discussion point

A paramedic delivers a patient with a painful ankle to the triage nurse in the ED and asks the nurse if she can supply the patient with some Paracetamol. The nurse says she will need to seek a prescription from a doctor for this as she is not suitably qualified. The paramedic says she does not need to do that as the drug is GSL and anybody can administer it. Who is right and on what basis? What other option can be considered for administration of Paracetamol without a prescription?

Controlled drugs

One of the most common drugs to be given in paramedic practice is the POM exemption, Morphine. Morphine is a controlled drug and it was not until October 2003 that certain controlled drugs became available for use under PGD, though only for specified professionals, such as specially trained nurses in EDs and coronary care units (MHRA, 2010). Paramedics are not included in the specified groups and therefore continue to administer such drugs under POM exemption.

As a controlled drug, Morphine requires systems and policies that prevent its misuse. Whereas the MHRA holds overarching responsibility for legislation of most medicines, it is the Home Office that governs the use of all controlled drugs including those intended for medicinal purposes. 'Controlled drugs' are those that have the potential to cause significant harm if not used in the appropriate context. Drugs that fall into this category must be produced, stored, prescribed, supplied and administered under stringent controls and measures. The most important document that relates to the use of controlled drugs is the Misuse of Drugs Act of 1971, which details how controlled drugs should be managed in the clinical environment. However, within the original Act, there was no mention of the use of controlled drugs in the ambulance sector, a clinical development which did not begin until much later and was therefore addressed in subsequent legislation. It is only later legislation that specifically relates to paramedics and controlled drugs as shown in Box 8.4.

Box 8.4   Legislation that relates specifically to paramedic practice

- Misuse of Drugs Regulations (MDR) 2001

  Group licence to St John Ambulance paramedics 2007
  Group authority for the possession of controlled drugs (NHS ambulance trusts and paramedics employed) 2008
  Group authority for the possession of controlled drugs (registered paramedics) 2008

- Medicines Act, 1968

Of these, it is the Misuse of Drugs Regulations (2001) that allows paramedics to possess and supply controlled drugs to any person who may lawfully possess them. The relevant group authority only applies for the immediate necessary treatment of sick or injured persons, as discussed previously, and when the individual is acting in his capacity as a paramedic.

Classification of controlled drugs

Controlled drugs are classified according to the following system, based on how harmful the drug can be if misused:

Class A
These are considered the most potentially harmful of the controlled drugs and include drugs such as Morphine, Diamorphine, Methadone, Ecstasy and Cocaine.
Class B
These are considered less harmful and include Cannabis, amphetamines and Codeine. If injected, some of these drugs become re-categorised as Class A.
Class C
These are considered the least harmful and include the benzodiazepines.

In addition, these drugs are further subdivided by 'schedule'; schedule 1 demanding the highest level of control and schedule 5 the lowest. Schedule

1 drugs have no medical use and are not found in clinical practice. Ecstasy is one example. Because such drugs require a Home Office license for production, possession or supply, a paramedic who encounters such drugs in the course of patient care cannot take possession of these drugs unless it is for the purpose of destroying the drug or for the purpose of handing the drugs to a police officer.

Schedule 2 controlled drugs, such as Morphine, have strict regulations regarding their storage and should be kept in a locked cupboard within a locked cupboard. In paramedic practice, the ambulance itself may be considered to be one of the two 'locked cupboards' and it is for this reason that paramedics must be meticulous in keeping their vehicle safe. In all clinical environments, controlled drugs should be checked and administered by two suitably qualified clinicians and a register of stock and transactions must be maintained for at least 2 years, though up to 7 years is deemed better practice (Davies, 2011).

Schedule 3 controlled drugs include such drugs as Temazepam, Midazolam and Buprenorphine. These drugs generally require safe custody although there are exceptions such as Midazolam, which does not need to be locked in a controlled drug cupboard. In addition, schedule 3 drugs do not need to be recorded in a controlled drugs register and do not require a witness to their destruction.

Schedule 4 drugs include other Benzodiazepines and anabolic steroids. Anabolic steroids are currently growing in popularity amongst young men in the United Kingdom and the Advisory Council on the Misuse of Drugs (ACMD) has expressed growing concern in relation to their misuse (ACMD, 2010).

Schedule 5 drugs include those medicines which contain lesser amounts of controlled drugs such as the analgesic Codeine or low strengths of Morphine. Both of these groups require less stringent controls.

Safety and security of controlled drugs in practice

In the last decade, measures around the security, safe-keeping and monitoring of controlled drugs have become more stringent overall, largely as a result of one particularly high-profile legal case known as, 'The Shipman Inquiry' (http://www.shipman-inquiry.org.uk). This case involved a GP, Harold Shipman, who, through a lack of checking and control, was able to unlawfully kill 15 patients through the administration of excess amounts of Morphine. He was found guilty of murder in his trial in the year 2000 and sentenced to life imprisonment. A number of inquiries subsequently took place in which it was postulated that Dr Shipman may in fact have unlawfully killed many more people, possibly as many as 200 (Dimond, 2012). As a GP, he often attended patients alone and he was in a position to issue death certificates and assert no need for an autopsy on his patients.

The Accountable Officer

As a result of lessons learned specifically from the fourth Shipman inquiry (DH, 2004), the additional measures put into place include the requirement for every applicable organisation to have in post an 'Accountable Officer' to take responsibility for the management of controlled drugs within their organisation. This includes the requirement for the Accountable Officer to share information and intelligence with a local intelligence network. An 'integrated and multidisciplinary inspectorate' was also recommended to monitor and audit all aspects of controlled drug usage from prescription to disposal. The necessity for a complete audit trail was identified so that controlled drug usage could be clearly tracked at every stage of its journey from pharmacy to patient's home or hospital bed. Every organisation will have its own procedures for reporting and investigating any inaccuracies relating to controlled drugs and it is each individual healthcare professional's responsibility to be aware of these.

An important role of the Accountable Officer is to ensure the adequate destruction and disposal arrangements of controlled drugs (Dimond, 2012). Any controlled drugs that have expired must be destroyed and this must be witnessed by an authorised individual who has been appointed by the Trust's Accountable officer. Disposal of controlled drugs can clearly be problematic in the pre-hospital environment and this was also highlighted in the Shipman enquiry. Dr Shipman exploited situations where patients had died at home and had perhaps been in medical need of a syringe driver containing controlled drugs. The informal custom was for District Nurses to subsequently remove such drugs and equipment but if no District Nurse was present, it was feasible for Dr Shipman (or indeed anyone else) to remove the drugs for his own intentions. Since paramedics in particular are sometimes called to the home of a terminally ill patient who has died, they need to be aware of the potential for misuse of drugs in this situation.

Part doses of controlled drugs that have not been administered to patients may also need to be disposed of either in the home or in hospital and this should be done safely and according to best practice. Downie et al. (2008) suggest that small quantities of controlled drugs can be flushed down a sink with running water to render them irretrievable. However, Water UK (2011, p. 13) states that,

'There is well documented evidence to show that the pharmaceutically active products in hospital waste water can be detected in the effluent from sewage treatment works and aquatic ecosystems. Once in the aquatic environment there is the potential for harm to living organisms including humans. It is imperative that robust waste arrangements are in place to ensure correct disposal of waste medication to prevent the discharge of harmful pharmaceuticals into the environment'.

Water UK (2011) goes on to assert that only non-pharmaceutically active medications such as glucose solution, normal saline and liquid nutritional feeds may be discharged into a sink, in small quantities of up to 1 l.

The denaturing of controlled drugs for safe disposal is considered to be best practice. Denaturing involves physically mixing the medicines with a binding matrix to make the material physically irretrievable in the waste chain (Environment Agency, 2010). Denaturing kits provide a safe, easy and reliable way to deactivate and make safe un-needed controlled drugs. Once denatured or rendered irretrievable, a controlled drug ceases to be classified. Accidental breakage of a controlled drug ampoule should be treated and recorded in a similarly formal way and every healthcare professional should know the policy and procedures in his or her own Trust.

A recent scoping exercise commissioned by the Department of Health and produced by the National Prescribing Centre (NPC, 2012) in collaboration with the National Institute for Health and Clinical Excellence (NICE) has identified that a small number of operational personnel within the ambulance and paramedic sector may not have a good understanding of the legislation relating to the management of medicines generally, and of controlled drugs in particular. Within the scoping exercise, the Ambulance Pharmacists' Network, a group of specialist pharmacists who advise NHS ambulance trusts on medicines management and legal and professional compliance, has also raised issues such as inconsistencies in controlled drug regulation and has sought clarification on the interpretation of controlled drug legislation.

In the exercise, front-line practitioners and senior managers identified areas of confusion around maximum dosages of Morphine that are permitted for use in paramedic practice and also around the use of different formulations of Diazepam (rectal and intravenous). As a result of misinterpreting legislation based on the 2008 group authority for the possession of controlled drugs, some ambulance Trusts had developed PGDs for rectal Diazepam when this was not in fact necessary. However, this particular legislation applies only to paramedics, therefore in situations where a nurse works for the ambulance service, a PGD would be needed for the administration of rectal Diazepam by that nurse.

The scoping exercise also identified that ambulance Trusts did not always understand that PGDs are not required for POM exemption drugs. It is also not necessary to have PGDs for the administration of non-parenteral POMs although it was acknowledged that some Trusts did this as matter of governance. As a result of this scoping exercise, the following three recommendations have been made.

Recommendation 1

The Home Office should consider clarifying the group authority and Misuse of Drug Regulations for the possession and administration of CDs, to prevent inconsistent and incorrect interpretations.

Recommendation 2

The Home Office should provide clarification on:

- The diazepam formulations that are included in the group authority.
- The maximum amount of morphine sulphate that may be administered to one person at any time and whether this could be increased to suit particular clinical circumstances.

Recommendation 3

The Home Office should consider amending the Misuse of Drugs Regulations to authorise NHS health professionals who can administer and supply CDs under PGD to lawfully possess the medicine for the purposes described within the PGD. This would allow nurses to provide the same level of service as paramedics, working within the same role as Emergency Care Practitioners (National Prescribing Centre, provided by NICE, 2012).

The majority of medicines used in emergency care are not controlled drugs. However, this does not mean that healthcare professionals can be complacent about their use and management. All drugs should be appropriately stored and managed, according to local policy and procedure.

Discussion point

A paramedic/technician crew attend a patient with cardiac chest pain. The paramedic administers 7.5 mg of Morphine for pain relief in the patient's home. The paramedic then asks the technician to go and bring the carry chair in and at the same time, to destroy the remaining 2.5 mg of Morphine in the ambulance. The paramedic says he will have to remain with the patient due to his clinical status and administration of Morphine. Under what legal condition has the Morphine been administered? What is the correct course of action for dealing with the remaining 2.5 mg Morphine? And what should the technician do in order to maintain legal and professional requirements?

Joint Royal Colleges Liaison Committee

Paramedic practice is largely influenced by the work and recommendations of the Joint Royal Colleges Liaison Committee (JRCALC). JRCALC is an important body comprising members from both the ambulance service and various organisations that have a professional concern in relation to what happens in emergency care and pre-hospital care. Largely medically dominated, many of the local decisions regarding drug protocols derive from the JRCALC guidelines (JRCALC, 2006) and these are duly adapted and applied by the various different ambulance Trusts up and down the country. This accounts for the degree of regional variation regarding which drugs paramedics can administer. Locally, this is done by means of an agreed formulary which is a range of drugs agreed on by the key stakeholders in that particular area, but which must be based on the larger JRCALC formulary. Interestingly, these guidelines do not cover the governance and safer management of controlled drugs.

Decisions as to what drugs go into a local formulary may be made on issues such as training needs associated with particular drugs or on cost. Downie et al. (2008) suggest that a formulary is an essential element in the drive to achieve safe and rational prescribing, and therefore, by inference, an essential element in the end point of administration. Formularies can be unpopular with independent prescribers because they restrict clinical freedom, patient choice and treatment options (Downie et al., 2008). However, this is currently of little consequence to the paramedic. From a paramedic perspective, the advantages of formularies outweigh the disadvantages because they allow greater treatment options on scene, in a relatively safe protocol-led environment. Given that there is currently no definitive move towards paramedic prescribing and the educational component of a paramedic's education is currently minimal in most curricula, this provides an important safeguard for both patient and paramedic.

Professional accountability in medicines management

The accountability of all registered healthcare professionals demands that great care is taken to administer the correct drug, in the correct form, in the correct dose, to the correct person, at the correct time, by the correct method. In addition, the clinician must be able to undertake an appropriate patient history and reach a reasoned and logical decision regarding treatment options, by deciding on the nature of the presenting complaint and how best to manage it. In doing so, they should reach the correct clinical decision regarding the necessity for drug intervention. Once a course of treatment involving drug therapy is reached, they must be able to articulate to the patient the risks and benefits associated with the medication and to consequently seek informed consent. Informed patient consent requires this information, and also that the patient is capable of understanding it, before consent can be rendered valid (Clark et al., 2012).

Despite the many safeguards associated with medicine administration, errors do still occur are sometimes the subject of 'fitness to practice' hearings under standards set by the governing bodies of each profession. For nurses, this is the Nursing and Midwifery Council (NMC) but for the allied health professions, the HCPC presides over such standards. 'Fitness to practice' refers to a practitioner's suitability to be on the register, with no restrictions (Griffith and Tangney, 2010). An example of a restriction might be that following an investigation and hearing, the professional body might impose a sanction that no longer allows a particular practitioner to work with medicines in an unsupervised fashion. Depending on the nature and circumstances of an error, the governing body may revoke the practitioner's registration, effectively 'striking them off'.

Medication errors can be irretrievable in terms of harm to the patient and also to the practitioner's career. To avoid such errors, practitioners should follow the standard checking procedure for any drug and document it accordingly. To help with this, the Medicines Act (1968) describes the information that must be available on any medication packaging. This includes the name of the product (by either its approved name or a proprietary name); the pharmaceutical form (tablet, capsule, injection, syrup); the strength of the product; the quantity in the package (e.g. the number of tablets); any special storage instructions; the method or route of administration; the batch number and expiry date. It is the practitioner's responsibility to check these carefully before administering any drug. Shortcuts should never be taken, even in the most dire of emergencies. Documentation should be precise and contemporaneous as well as unambiguous and, if not electronically generated, legible. It is also equally important to document if medication, e.g. analgesia, has been offered but refused by the patient. This demonstrates that the practitioner has considered appropriate treatments within his duty of care to the patient even though the patient may have declined those treatments. Documentation can and may be used in both fitness to practice hearings and in courts of law. It will either support or condemn the practitioner (Griffith and Tangney, 2010) and it is equally important to remember that if something has not been documented then in the eyes of the law, it has not been done (Gawthorpe, 2010).

It is a professional responsibility to report any errors or incidents involving medication or medical devices. Incidents involving medical devices are generally explored and investigated by the MHRA with a view to learning lessons and sharing those lessons with the wider professions. Every organisation will have its own policy and procedure for reporting errors and incidents. Significant numbers of medication errors occur each year and in an 18-month period spanning 2005–2006, over 60,000 incidents were reported to the National Patient Safety Agency (NPSA, 2007). The NPSA is an arm's-length body of the Department of Health and works in tandem with the

MHRA, operating the National Reporting and Learning Service (NRLS). The NPSA encourages staff and indeed the public to report incidents, including 'near misses', via its online reporting system. This information is rendered anonymous and subsequently, data and incidents are analysed by experts in order to identify hazards, risks and opportunities to improve the safety of patient care. Learning points are disseminated to healthcare organisations via the development of tools and specific guidance at a local level. In fact, anyone with an NHS email address can log into the system and review incidents and outcomes relating to their own Trusts.

The roles and organisation of arm's-length bodies like the National Patient Safety Agency are presently subject to some reform as a result of government policy (DH, 2010b). As a result, some may merge with others, some may be disbanded and some may change their function. Therefore, the information presented in this part of the chapter may change in the near future but the important underlying principles of reporting and investigating drug errors with a view to managing patient safety and educating staff will remain.

Because of the nature of paramedic practice in particular, where there is often only one or two practitioners present, it is possible to covertly manage an error involving medication. It is the integrity of the individual/individuals involved that will determine whether or not this occurs. One small-scale study (Vilke et al., 2007) reported that about 1 in 10 of 352 paramedics who were surveyed admitted to a medication error during a 1-year period and that 4% of these errors were not formally reported. The errors mainly concerned dose-related errors, protocol errors, wrong route and wrong medication errors. Contributing factors were said to include failure to check the medicine and infrequent use of particular medicines.

A registered professional is required to demonstrate honesty and integrity in everything that he or she does and to uphold the public's confidence in the profession (NMC, 2008; HCPC, 2012). The ethics of a situation and the moral values of each practitioner will influence their actions and can present the practitioner with an uncomfortable dilemma. Lawson and Hennefer (2010) define an ethical dilemma as a situation in which there are at least two ways in which a practitioner might respond and of these two ways,

- neither option is entirely satisfactory
- there is a clash of values
- the options themselves appear impossible

Ethics in healthcare is understood to pertain to the collective beliefs of a community whereas morals involve a more personal stance (Gawthorpe, 2010) (see further information in Chapter 6). It is the duty of all practitioners to protect the patient whilst improving medication safety in whatever ways they can. Therefore, there should be a moral and ethical obligation to report any medication errors, no matter the circumstances. Furthermore, non-adherence to the either the Medicines Act or the Misuse of Drugs Act renders the practitioner accountable by law for committing a criminal act.

Continuous professional development

It is important for all healthcare professionals to keep abreast of changes in legislation and clinical practice relating to medicines and their management. For example, it is possible for drugs to change their status from POM to pharmacy or GSL medicines, often in response to societal need. Recent examples of medicines that were formerly POM include emergency contraception and nicotine replacement therapy. A clinical example of the importance of keeping up to date with regard to drug administration is the change in best practice for intramuscular injection of drugs in recent years (Doherty and Lister, 2011). Anecdotal evidence suggests that many clinicians remain unaware of the ventrogluteal site as the site with least risk of complications for intramuscular injection and continue to routinely use sites such as the deltoid muscle or the lateral aspect of the thigh for this purpose. Whilst these sites are not inherently wrong, neither are they best practice, and consequently the clinician should be able to justify the use of other sites, if challenged to do so.

In respect of the paramedic role, with its rapid rate of development, it may be time to consider the degree of taught pharmacology within paramedic curricula. Since the opening of the HPC (now HCPC) Paramedic Register in 2003, there has been a mass movement towards higher education for paramedic practice. It could be argued that in order to be safe in drug administration, a paramedic practitioner requires knowledge of drug absorption mechanisms; the metabolic action of the liver; the excretory function of the kidneys, as well as the effects and side effects of drugs that they will commonly use or encounter. This has to be balanced against the requirement to turn out a competent paramedic with the relevant clinical skills and under pinning knowledge in sometimes in as little as 2 years on a diploma programme. This is quite a challenge and does strengthen the argument for an all degree profession which is now the case for the majority of healthcare professionals.

Sources of drug information

Until such times, Gregory and Ward (2010) recommend five good sources of drug information for paramedics which are:

- The Joint Royal Colleges Ambulance Liaison Committee (JRCALC)
- The British National Formulary (BNF)
- Medication Package inserts

- National Poisons Information Service
- Pharmacology textbooks.

With the exception of the JRCALC, all will have similar relevance to any practitioner working in emergency or urgent care (with the exception of the JRCALC). All healthcare professional should additionally be aware of the NICE in relation to its role in recommending the drugs that are considered best options for clinical use. Guidelines produced by NICE should be adhered to by all healthcare organisations.

Summary

This chapter has highlighted the necessity for healthcare professionals to be aware of the legislation surrounding medicines and their management. The different methods by which medicines are administered in the emergency and urgent care arena have been explored, including the use of POM exemptions, medicines which can be administered by anyone for the purpose of saving a life and PGDs. Progress on the issue of prescribing for paramedics has been raised, as well as potential changes to the legislation surrounding paramedic students and the administration of parenteral drugs during their training periods. An explanation of the clinical issues surrounding controlled drugs and their different classifications has been provided and the uppermost responsibility of the accountable practitioner has been stressed. It is largely through continuous professional development and reflection (see Chapter 5 for further detail) in each individual, accountable practitioner that medicines management will be made safer for the patient.

References

Advisory Council on the Misuse of Drugs (ACMD) (2010) *Consideration of the Anabolic Steroids*. Available at http://webarchive. nationalarchives.gov.uk/+/http://www.homeoffice.gov.uk/publications/ drugs/acmd1/anabolic-steroids-report/anabolic-steroids?view=Binary (accessed 8 June 2012).

Association of Ambulance Chief Executives (2011) *Taking Healthcare to the Patient 2: A Review of 6 Years' Progress and Recommendations for the Future*. Available at www.ambulanceleadershipforum.com (accessed 8 June 2012).

Axe, S. (2011) Issues for debate: numeracy and nurse prescribing: do the standards achieve their aim? *Nurse Education in Practice*, **11**(5), 285–287.

Broadhead, R. (2011) Professional, legal and ethical issues in relation to prescribing practice. In: *The Textbook of Non-Medical Prescribing* (eds D. Nutall & J. Rutt-Howard). Wiley Blackwell, Chichester.

Clark, V., Harris, G. & Cowland, S. (2012) Ethics and law for the paramedic. In: *Foundations for Paramedic Practice*, 2nd edn (ed. A. Blaber). McGraw Hill Education, Berkshire.

College of Paramedics (2011a) *Paramedic Exemption Medicines & Pre-registered Student Paramedics*. Available at https://www.collegeofparamedics.co.uk/news/archive/2011/08/08/paramedic_exemption_medicines_pre-registered _student_paramedics (accessed 2 June 2012).

College of Paramedics (2011b) *An Important Update on Paramedic Exemption Medicines and Pre-registered Student Paramedics*. Available at https://www.collegeofparamedics.co.uk/news/archive/2011/08/29/an_ important_update_on_paramedic_exemption_medicines_pre-registered_ student (accessed 2 June 2010).

Colleen, A. (2012) Medicines and Prescribing Update *College of Paramedics Newsletter*, **2**(4), 3.

Courtenay, M. & Griffiths, M. (2007) Implementation across the United Kingdom. In: *Non-Medical Prescribing in Health Care Practice – A Toolkit for Students and Practitioners* (eds D. Brookes & A. Smith). Palgrave MacMillan, Basingstoke.

Davies, J. (2011) Legislation surrounding the administration of medicines by paramedics. *Journal of Paramedic Practice*, **3**(8), 424–428.

Department of Health (DH) (1999) *Review of Prescribing, Supply and Administration of medicines – Final Report*. Available at http://www.dh.gov.uk/prod_consum_dh/groups/dh_digitalassets/@dh/@en/documents/digitalasset/dh_4077153.pdf (accessed 31 May 2012).

Department of Health (DH) (2001) *Reforming Emergency Care*, Department of Health, London.

Department of Health (DH) (2004) *Shipman Inquiry Fourth Report: The Regulation of Controlled Drugs in the Community*. Available at http://www.shipman-inquiry.org.uk/images/fourthreport/SHIP04_COMPLETE_NO_APPS.pdf (accessed 2 June 2012).

Department of Health (DH) (2005) *Taking Healthcare to the Patient, Transforming NHS Ambulance Services*, Department of Health, London.

Department of Health (DH) (2010a) *Proposals to Introduce Prescribing Responsibilities for Paramedics: Stakeholder Engagement*. Available at http://www.dh.gov.uk/en/Publicationsandstatistics/Publications/PublicationsPolicyAnd Guidance/DH_114355 (accessed 2 June 2012).

Department of Health (DH) (2010b) *Reforming Arm's Length Bodies*. Available at http://www.direct.gov.uk/prod_consum_dg/groups/dg_digitalas sets/@dg/@en/documents/digitalasset/dg_186443.pdf (accessed 8 June 2012).

Dimond, B. (2012) *Legal Aspects of Medicines*, 2nd edn. Quay Books, London.

Doherty, L. & Lister, S. (2011) (eds) *The Royal Marsden Hospital Manual of Clinical Nursing*, Procedures 8th edn. Wiley Blackwell, Oxford.

Downie, G., Mackenzie, J., Williams, A. & Hind, C. (2008) *Pharmacology and Medicines management for Nurses*, 4th edn. Elsevier, Edinburgh.

Doy, R. & Turner, K. (2004) The giraffe: the emergency care practitioner; fit for purpose? The East Anglian experience. *Emergency Medicine Journal*, **21**, 365–366.

Eastwood, K., Boyle, M. & Williams, B. (2009) Mathematical and drug calculation abilities of paramedic students. *Emergency Medicine Journal*. doi: 10.1136/emj.2008.070789.

Eastwood, K., Boyle, M. & Williams, B. (2011a) Can paramedics accurately perform drug calculations? *Emergency Medicine Journal*, **26**, 117–118.

Eastwood, K., Boyle, M., Williams, B. & Fairhall, R. (2011b) Numeracy skills of nursing students. *Nurse Education Today*, **31**(8), 815–818.

Environment Agency (2010) *Denaturing of Controlled drugs at a Place Other than the Premises of production – Regulatory Position Statement*. Available at http://www.environment-agency.gov.uk/static/documents/Business/MWRP_RPS_004_v2_denaturing_drugs_final_08-07-10.pdf (accessed 2 June 2012).

Gawthorpe, D. (2010) The law governing medicines. In: *Medicines Management in Adult Nursing* (eds L. Lawson & D. Hennefer), pp 63–79. Learning Matters, Exeter.

Gregory, P. & Ward, A. (2010) *Sanders Paramedic Textbook*. Mosby Elsevier, Edinburgh.

Griffith, G. & Tangney, C. (2010) *Law and Professional Issues in Nursing*. 2nd edn. Learning Matters, Exeter.

Health & Care Professions Council (2012) *Standards of Conduct, Performance and Ethics*. HCPC, London.

Joint Royal Colleges Ambulance Liaison Committee (JRCALC) (2006) *JRCALC Guidelines*. Available at http://www2.warwick.ac.uk/fac/med/research/hsri/emergencycare/prehospitalcare/jrcalcstakeholderwebsite/guidelines (accessed 2 June 2012).

Lawson, E. & Hennefer, D. (2010) Partnership working. In: *Medicines Management in Adult Nursing* (eds E. Lawson & D. Hennefer). Learning Matters, Exeter.

McMullan, M., Jones, R. & Lea, S. (2010) Patient safety: numerical skills and drug calculation abilities of nursing students and registered nurses. *Journal of Advanced Nursing*, **66**(4), 891–899.

McQueen, D., Begg, M. & Maxwell, S. (2010) eDrugCalc: an online self-assessment package to enhance medical students' drug dose calculation skills. *British Journal of Clinical Pharmacology*, **70**(4), 492-499.

Medicines Act (1968) Great Britain (1968) Medicines Act 1968. Available at http://www.legislation.gov.uk/ukpga/1968/67 12 June 2012 (accessed 12 June 2012).

Medicines Healthcare Regulation Agency (MHRA) (2003) *Letter to Interested Parties – Administration of Medicines by Ambulance Paramedics: Amendment to the Prescription Only Medicines (Human use) Order 1997*. Available at http://www.mhra.gov.uk/SearchHelp/GoogleSearch/index.htm?q=www.mhra.gov.uk%2Fhome%2Fgroups%2Fcomms-ic%2F...%2Fcon007636.doc (accessed 12 June 2012).

Medicines Healthcare Regulation Agency (MHRA) (2005) *Paramedics: Exemptions*. Available at http://www.mhra.gov.uk/Howweregulate/Medicines/Availabilityprescribingsellingandsupplyingofmedicines/ExemptionsfromMedicinesActrestrictions/Paramedics/index.htm (accessed 2 June 2012).

Medicines Healthcare Regulation Agency (MHRA) (2010) *Exemptions for Parenteral Administration in an Emergency to Human Beings of Certain Prescription Only Medicines*. Available at http://www.mhra.gov.uk/home/groups/es-policy/documents/publication/con096764.pdf (accessed 8 June 20120).

Misuse of Drugs Act (1971) Great Britain (1971) Misuse of Drugs Act 1971. Available at http://www.legislation.gov.uk/ukpga/1971/38/contents (accessed 12 June 2012).

Misuse of Drugs Regulations (2001) Great Britain (2001) Misuse of Drugs Regulations 2001. Available at http://www.legislation.gov.uk/uksi/2001/3998/contents/made (accessed 10 June 2012).

National Patient Safety Agency (2007) *Safety in Doses: Medication Safety Incidents in the NHS*. Available at http://www.nrls.npsa.nhs.uk/EasySiteWeb/getresource.axd?AssetID=61392 (accessed 17 July 2012).

National Prescribing Centre (NPC) (2009) *Patient Group Directions – a Practical Guide and Framework of Competencies for all Professionals using Patient Group Directions*. Available at http://www.somed.org/members/ITstudentinfo/ITinfo9.pdf (accessed 12 June 2012).

National Prescribing Centre provided by NICE (2012) *Safe Management and Use of Controlled Drugs in the Ambulance and Paramedic Services in England*. Available at http://www.npc.nhs.uk/controlled_drugs/resources/final_reports/final_report_safe_management_and_use_of_controlled_drugs_in_the_ambulance_and_paramedic_services_in_england.pdf (accessed 2 June 2012).

North West Ambulance Service (NWAS) (2009) *Drug Administration Protocol Reference Guide*. North West Ambulance Service. Bolton.

Nursing and Midwifery Council (NMC) (2008) *The Code: Standards for Conduct, Performance and Ethics*, NMC, London.

Nursing and Midwifery Council (NMC) (2010) *Standards for the Administration of Medicines*. Available at http://www.nmc-uk.org/Documents/Standards/nmcStandardsForMedicinesManagementBooklet.pdf (accessed 12 June 2012).

Prescription Only Medicine (Human Use) Order (1997) Available at http://www.legislation.gov.uk/uksi/2003/696/pdfs/uksi_20030696_en.pdf (accessed 12 June 2012).

Royal College of Nursing (2004) *Patient Group Directions – Guidance and information for Nurses*. Royal College of Nursing, London.

Tinson, S. (2007) Government targets – getting the best from non-medical prescribing. In: *Non-Medical Prescribing in Health Care Practice – A Toolkit for Students and Practitioners* (eds D. Brookes & A. Smith). Palgrave MacMillan, Basingstoke.

Royal Pharmaceutical Society (2004) *Omeprazole Quick Reference Guide*. Available at www.rpharms.com (accessed 12 June 2012).

Vilke, G., Tornaben, S., Stepanski, B., Shipp, H., Ray, L., Metz, M. et al (2007) Paramedic Self-reported Medication Errors. *Prehospital Emergency Care*, **11**(1), 80–84.

Water UK (2011) *National Guidance for Healthcare Waste Water Discharges*. Available at http://www.water.org.uk/home/policy/publications/archive/industry-guidance/wastewater-from-hospitals/national-guidance-hospital-discharges-april-2011-v1.pdf?s1=controlled&s2=drugs (accessed 8 June 2012).

Websites

National Electronic Library for Medicines. Available at http://www.
  nelm.nhs.uk
National Patient Safety Agency. Available at http://www.npsa.nhs.uk/
Skills for Health. Available at www.skillsforhealth.org.uk.
The Shipman Inquiry. Available at http://www.shipman-inquiry.org.uk

9 Continuing Professional Development and Portfolio Development

Val Nixon

Faculty of Health Sciences, Staffordshire University, Stafford, UK

Introduction

The political agenda in the late 1990s set out to modernise the national health service (NHS) through implementation of national quality standards. To ensure local delivery, the clinical governance agenda acknowledged that lifelong learning and continuous professional development (CPD) for all healthcare professionals was fundamental to deliver national quality standards. CPD is now a legal requirement for all health professionals to continue on the professional register and are required to maintain a professional portfolio to record all their CPD activities.

This chapter offers a brief overview of the political and professional drivers that led to the importance and development of lifelong learning and CPD. It is not the intention to explore the detailed requirements of regulatory body standards for CPD and renewal of registration as these are easily accessible from the regulatory organisations. However, a brief summary of the professional requirements will be given to introduce the link with CPD and professional portfolios. An introduction of portfolios will begin with a definition of an educational versus a professional portfolio, but professional portfolios will be the main focus of discussion as it is beyond the remit of this chapter to explore educational portfolios in greater depth. Nevertheless, while the aims of the educational and professional portfolios will differ, the principles of the professional portfolio will have many similarities to the educational portfolio.

Most healthcare professionals make the assumption that CPD involves attending and completing courses, which is not entirely true. CPD involves a range of activities that are appropriate to personal and professional

Professional Practice in Paramedic, Emergency and Urgent Care, First Edition. Edited by Val Nixon.
© 2013 John Wiley & Sons, Ltd. Published 2013 by John Wiley & Sons, Ltd.

development and these will be introduced how to plan activities and organise them in a structured professional portfolio.

Many healthcare professionals are unsure of the practical issues relating
to the development of portfolios and they also tend to attach a tenuous
link between the documentation in portfolios and portfolio learning. This
chapter will therefore offer a practical guide and examples on how to
compile a professional portfolio. This will include self-assessment tools,
various forms of evidence to include; organisation and structure of a
portfolio.

Continuous professional development

The New NHS: Modern Dependable (Department of Health (DH), 1997) targeted professional educational bodies to continue to develop an infrastruc-
ture for CPD. Two years later in 1999, the introduction of a First Class Service (DH) proposed to deliver a consistent approach to high-quality care
through the implementation of national quality standards such as National
Service Frameworks (NSFs) and the National Institute for Clinical Excellence (NICE). As a consequence, clinical governance was introduced to provide a mechanism to ensure local delivery of high-quality clinical services
which was supported through programmes of lifelong learning and professional self-regulation (DH, 1999). Gopee (2008) claims that the concept of
lifelong learning has been examined with intense attention since the 1970s;
however, the realisation of this concept as 'an investment in quality' (DH,
1997) and investment in staff (DH, 2000) led to an increasing recognition of
lifelong learning and CPD over the past decade.

The NHS must keep pace with a changing world, medical advances, fast
changing new technologies and new approaches in order to deliver a high-
quality patient care. Greater public awareness of these advances has rightly
created increased expectations of what the NHS should deliver and have a
right to access quality healthcare provided by skilled and knowledgeable
healthcare practitioners. In addition, the development and complexity of
organisations continually demand a wider range of skills from practitioners. These increasing demands require efficient, supported and structured
development for CPD (Royal College of Nursing (RCN), 2007).

Politically, CPD and lifelong learning are about growth and opportunity, about making sure that individuals, teams and organisations have the
knowledge and skills that can help shape and change things for the better,
improving the patient experience and thus essential to the future quality of
the health service (Draper and Clark, 2007). Furthermore, it enables professionals to expand and fulfil their potential (DH, 1997). At a practice level,
CPD is a term given to learning and development which takes place in
a professional's career after the point of qualification and/or registration.
Nurses and paramedics are required by law to undertake CPD to maintain

competence in order to re-register with their regulatory bodies. This is to ensure that they continue to learn and develop throughout their careers and are able to work safely, legally and effectively (Health & Care Professions Council, 2012a) and to:

- provide a high standard of practice and care
- keep up to date with new developments in practice
- think and reflect for themselves
- demonstrate that they are keeping up to date and developing practice

(Nursing and Midwifery Council (NMC), 2011)

An important principle of CPD is that it includes much more than going on courses. There are a range of formal and informal activities which health professionals maintain and develop professional and personal knowledge, skills and competences (see Table 9.1). It is important to note that an increasingly large proportion of CPD is work based and all health organisations need to develop a learning culture and create a learning environment. In addition, CPD should also reflect a responsible and proactive approach to one's own on-going professional learning and requires a personal pledge to lifelong learning in order to maintain, improve or develop new competence within their professional role.

The activities outlined in Table 9.1 which you may undertake during your professional career are varied to demonstrate your personal and professional development. It is important that these activities are relevant to your professional role, demonstrate application of theory to practice, and that you can show what you have learned from it. Your CPD should reflect a cross section of the activities and should demonstrate your learning and development and the impact this has had on your professional role.

Table 9.1   Examples of CPD activities

Formal learning	Informal
Attending workshops, conferences, courses	Reviewing books and journals
	Case studies
Undertaking project work	Reflective practice
Writing for publication	Clinical supervision
Undertaking research study	Discussions with colleagues
Mentoring students	Shadowing senior colleagues
Developing and implementing policies, protocols, guidelines	Critical incident analysis
	Writing narratives/stories
Role expansion	Chairing meetings
Undertaking clinical audits	Group membership of steering groups, working groups etc.

> **Discussion point**
>
> Communication skills, leadership qualities and abilities, theoretical understandings of professional, legal and ethical principles are knowledge – skills and competences required in most aspects of our personal, professional role. Consider areas of your development for these skills and identify what activities would be most suited to supporting your progression and development.

CPD should be planned rather than a random collection of activities undertaken as and when convenient. In planning appropriate CPD, emphasis should be on the purpose and aim of activities together with the outcomes in terms of the skills development and additional knowledge that you will gain. The HCPC and NMC requirements are for health professionals to maintain a current and accurate record of their CPD activities. This can be recorded in whatever format is most convenient; however, both regulatory bodies can request this to be a written professional portfolio to explain how you demonstrate to keep up to date with practice to meet their required standards (NMC, 2011; HCPC, 2012a). (For further details on the standards for CPD and renewal of registration, go to www.hcpc-org.uk and www.nmc-uk.org.)

What is a professional portfolio?

Portfolios are commonly referred to as an 'educational portfolio' or a 'professional portfolio'. An educational portfolio is used as an assessment strategy to measure the quality and quantity of student learning, progression and achievement. As an assessment strategy, the portfolio will contain a variety of information that can be used as evidence towards achievement of learning outcomes and therefore structured around a course or module. Baume (2001, p1) defines an education portfolio as

'a structured collection comprising of labelled evidence and critical reflection on that evidence ... it is presented to show evidence of that learning. It may additionally compose an explicit claim or demonstration that specified outcomes have been achieved'.

In contrast, a professional portfolio is a mandatory requirement to fulfil the regulatory body requirements and therefore the evidence and structure will focus around the personal and professional development and key attributes for a professional role. One of the most quoted definitions of portfolios is by Brown (1992, p. 1) who states that a portfolio is

'a private collection of evidence which demonstrates the continuing acquisition of skills, knowledge, understanding and achievement. It is both retrospective and prospective, as well as reflecting the current stage of development and activity of the individual'.

This would suggest that a portfolio can contain material from a variety of sources chosen by the individual as it is designed and constructed to portray a picture of its creator. Brown (1992, p. 1) claims that it is a 'private collection of evidence'; however, it is likely to be open to public scrutiny in some form as it may be used to demonstrate to others the quality of the work you have been doing. It provides a clear and concise framework within which a comprehensive resource can be built up that will be useful in a variety of ways including:

- Applying for a new post
- Compiling a curriculum vitae
- Seeking accreditation for prior learning and experience
- Participating in performance review
- Building a personal development profile
- Meeting the statutory requirements for renewing professional registration
- Evidence of competence against the NHS Knowledge and Skills Framework for NHS employees (DH, 2004)

(Nixon, 2008)

Foremost, among the many benefits for the portfolio, it allows the healthcare professional to be accountable and autonomous learners responsible for the direction and quality of their learning and professional development progress (Harris et al., 2001; Cangelosi, 2008). The potential of the portfolio depends upon the commitment of the individual, the value that is placed on its contents and regarding it as an essential part for his/her development (Jasper, 1995).

A professional portfolio will be your personal record of your achievements and there is a range of evidence you can use within your portfolio such as:

- Curriculum vitae
- Personal statement
- Certificates of study days, workshops, courses, mandatory training
- Testimonials
- Job descriptions
- Self-assessments
- Work-based learning activities – writing and/or implementing policies, protocols and/or guidelines
- Reflective writing
- Critical incidents/case studies
- Performance appraisal reviews

- Feedback from mentoring students
- Teaching activities
- Project work

For many healthcare professionals, there is an expectation that the professional portfolio will incorporate reflective writing to demonstrate the individual's learning experience and the personal and professional development from that particular learning experience (reflection and reflective writing is discussed in detail in Chapter 5). Coffey (2005) suggests the collated evidence provides a 'series of snapshots' over time, which represent an individual's experiences and learning from and about practice.

Starting your portfolio

When starting your portfolio, it may seem a daunting task at first as it can be difficult to know where to start and what evidence to use. It would seem common sense to start putting in your curriculum vitae (CV), certificates of courses, workshops, testimonials, reflections and whatever other pieces of paper you can use to fill out your portfolio, yet, generally, portfolios tend to be unstructured and contain irrelevant evidence that does not demonstrate any achievements. One recurring finding in research examining users' experiences of portfolios is that clearer guidance on expected content and structure is needed in order to reduce inclusion of unnecessary evidence and increase the quality of evidence supporting claims for achievement in a given area of practice (Baume, 2001; Driessen et al., 2005; Rees et al., 2005; General Medical Council (GMC), 2007).

When starting your professional portfolio, it is important to remember that it is more than a *hodgepodge* of information and lists of professional activities. It is an organised collection of evidence detailing your specific accomplishments and what you have learnt from it and the critical starting point is effective planning for CPD. The purpose of this is to recognise through your self-assessment where you are now and where you want (and need) to be (Knowles et al., 2005) and how you will achieve and evaluate your development.

Self-assessment against professional development

Self-assessment occurs when you make judgements about aspects of your own performance and it is an important skill for lifelong learning (Boud, 1995). Self-assessment enables you to take responsibility for your own learning and will therefore allow you to take control and ownership of how you will meet your development needs (Stoker, 1998). It is necessary to monitor your performance and motivation needed to become an independent learner as lifelong learning requires that individuals should be able to work independently and assess their own performance and progress (Falchikov and Boud, 1989).

Self-assessment helps to identify strengths and gaps between your knowledge, skills and experience and consequently acts as a scaffold to build your portfolio. Each of us possesses certain strengths and weaknesses and it is very easy to assume that self-assessment is easy and that we are able to self-assess independently. For many of us though, knowing what we are best at and worst at does not necessarily come easily and generally we can overlook our strengths in favour of our weaknesses. Mattheos et al. (2004) claims that the ability to accurately self-assess competence and achievement is not a natural gift; however, the skills can be learned and improved, and thus, need to be facilitated (Boud, 1992). The importance of being motivated to take ownership and investment in your personal and professional development cannot be over-emphasized and having the skills to undertake your self-assessment will help to shift the focus from 'how good am I?' to 'how better can I get?' (Mattheos et al., 2004). At different stages in your professional career whether you are a novice or expert (Benner, 1984) you will have some clear ideas about some of your strengths and perhaps some of your weaker areas too. A good starting point is to pull together those ideas and list them in a SWOT analysis.

SWOT analysis

A SWOT is a simple tool to use to start your journey and is an acronym for *strengths, weaknesses, opportunities and threats*. Strengths and weaknesses are considered internal factors as this relates to you as an individual. When completing these sections you should be able to list your personal qualities, study habits, your knowledge and skills gained through personal and professional development. Opportunities and threats are considered external factors that can enable or obstruct your development. The key is to identify those factors and use the opportunities to build on your strengths and to improve on your weaknesses and acknowledge your threats that will help you to develop strategies to overcome these. For example, if you record that dealing with bereaved relatives as a weakness, you may record communication skills as strength. Communication skills are fundamental when dealing with bereaved relatives, so you can use this strength to work towards addressing that particular weakness. Using that same weakness, threats such as limited exposure (when dealing with bereaved relatives) in pre-hospital setting, no local workshops and courses, unable to be released for study days etc., would inhibit your development. Yet, opportunities such as access to relevant distant learning courses, undertake a literature review, arrange to spend some time in a clinical areas such as Accident & Emergency departments and hospices are strategies you can use to overcome your threats and enable you to progress. It is useful to title your

SWOT analysis as you can write several that relate to different areas of development, such as clinical skills, caring for a particular group of patients, e.g. children and young adults, patients with mental health problems, career development for the next 5 years, or undertaking a new role. Box 9.1 gives an example of a completed SWOT analysis in relation to role development. Once you have completed your SWOT analysis, this will form the development of your goal(s) and actions you need to undertake for your development.

Box 9.1   Example of SWOT analysis (Evidence No. 4.1)

TITLE: SWOT analysis – To successfully undertake mentor role

STRENGTHS	WEAKNESSES
Good communication skills	Limited theoretical knowledge of learning styles and learning theories
Experienced paramedic with 6 years' experience	
Time management skills	Limited understanding of teaching and learning strategies
Very organised and good time management skills	Superficial knowledge of mentor role and responsibilities
Motivated and enthusiastic to learn	No previous experience of studying in higher education
Excellent IT skills	
Experience of supervising pre-registration students and newly qualified paramedics	No experience of academic writing skills
Teaching pre-registration students in practice	Presentation skills
Experience of facilitating clinical skills teaching in university	Lack of understanding of educational terminology, e.g. module outcomes, critical analysis, evaluation etc.
Good team player	Can be easily distracted
Can work well individually	Poor concentration
Recognise when support and guidance is needed	No knowledge of supporting students with learning disabilities
Knowledge of local policies, protocols and national guidelines	
Excellent knowledge of professional standards	
Providing peer support to colleagues	

OPPORTUNITIES	THREATS
To shadow mentors in practice	No students in clinical practice at the time of undertaking mentorship course
To undertake a mentorship course	
Gain experience of mentoring students in practice	No support from experienced mentors
Access to university library and library support	Time to attend study skills sessions
Study skills sessions	
IT support	Limited access to tutors
Peer support from experienced mentors in practice	No funding available to undertake mentorship course
Tutor support	No protected study time
Access to books, journals etc.	Lack of managerial support to develop mentor role
Development of presentation skills through mentorship course	Managing a difficult student in practice
Protected study time	Sickness

Goal setting and action plan

There are a plethora of self-assessment tools that can be of value towards making specific judgements about your performance and monitoring your progress. Self-assessment methods and tools can be varied within a portfolio and Boud (1992) describes a self-assessment regime in which you should undertake the following:

- Goal setting
- Specify the criteria that define whether those goals have been met
- Describe the evidence that would be presented claiming goals have been met
- Set out a case for claiming that the goals have been met
- Action plan

Bandura (1997) suggests that goals enhance self-regulation, through their effects on motivation, learning, self-efficacy (perceived capabilities for learning or performing actions at given levels), and self-evaluations of progress. Goals are involved across the different phases of self-regulation; planning (setting a goal and deciding on goal strategies); performance control (employing goal-directed actions and monitoring performance); and self-reflection (evaluating one's goal progress and adjusting strategies to ensure success) (Zimmerman, 1998).

Overall, goals are usually general intentions of what you want to do, abstract and difficult to validate, for example, 'to become an Emergency Care Practitioner in 5 years'. To achieve your overall goal, you would need to identify small steps to firm up into powerful, specific, precise goals (sometimes referred to as objectives) that are simple, concrete and easy to validate. For example, *'to complete an ECP course within 12 months', 'to increase my clinical experience of assessing and managing minor injuries'*, to *'develop theoretical knowledge of professional accountability'*.

When setting goals it is important not to set unrealistic, unachievable expectations and the use of the SMART is useful mnemonic to use to keep you on target. SMART usually stands for:

Specific – not 'wish lists' or vague statements
Measurable – do you know you are doing it and is it effective?
Achievable – do you have the resources to do it?
Realistic – is it possible?, can you deliver this?
Timely – when is it going to be done exactly?

Specific – Clear objectives that identify What, Why and How

- *What* are you going to do? Use action words such as direct, organize, coordinate, lead, develop, plan, build etc.
- *Why* is this important to do at this time? What do you want to ultimately accomplish?
- *How* are you going to do it?

If you set a precise goal by putting in dates, times and amounts so that achievement can be measured, then you know the exact objective to be achieved, and can take complete satisfaction from having completely achieved it. Goals that incorporate specific performance standards are more likely to enhance self-regulation and activate self-evaluations than general goals as 'do my best' or 'try hard' (Locke and Latham, 1990). Specific goals raise performance because they specify the amount of effort required for success and boost self-efficacy by providing a clear standard against which to determine progress. If you set yourself demanding goals and you are unable to achieve them, it is possible that you will feel frustrated and disappointed.

Measurable

When setting goals you would need to establish concrete evidence to measure your progression or achievement. For example, if your objective is to increase your knowledge on wound assessment, your evidence could be a reflective piece of writing or you may have a competency document provided by your trust. When you measure your progress, you stay on track, reach your target dates, and experience the exhilaration of achievement that spurs you on to continued effort required to reach your objective. If your objectives are so vague it can become useless and it is difficult to know whether you have achieved it. If achievement cannot be measured, then your self-confidence will not benefit, nor can you observe progress towards a greater goal. If you consistently fail to meet a measurable goal, then you can adjust it or analyse the reason for failure and take appropriate action to improve skills.

Achievable

When you identify goals that are most important to you, you begin to figure out ways you can make them come true and you identify previously overlooked opportunities to achieve them. Whilst you may start with the best intentions, goals that are far out of reach and not achievable will have an impact on your enthusiasm and self-determination to accomplish them and your ability to do your best will cease. For example, if your goal is to become an ECP in 5 years, you need to consider if the resources (ECP course and/or funding) exist and if the ambulance service or other NHS providers employ this role. If the resources are not available and the role does not exist in practice, then this will be unachievable. Consequently, this will dampen your enthusiasm, motivation and commitment to further your professional career. To make this achievable, you could change your goal to '*develop my professional, clinical knowledge and experience towards an advanced practitioner role*'. By changing your goal, this can be achievable as you could work towards expanding your role through clinical experience, gaining experience in Minor Injury Units and/or Accident and Emergency Departments, undertaking workshops that relate to assessment and management minor illnesses, injuries etc. This will not dampen your enthusiasm to progress in your career or restrict you to a specific role (that may not be achievable) and your objectives would be similar as mentioned above.

Relevant or realistic goals

This is not a synonym for 'easy'. Realistic, in this case means 'do-able'. Devise a plan or a way of getting there which makes the goal realistic. The goal needs to be realistic for you and where you are at the moment and it is important not to set goals too high or too low. When goals are set unrealistically high, it is perceived to be unreachable and no effort will be made to achieve it. Conversely, goals can be set so low that you feel no challenge of benefit in achieving the goal. Setting goals can seem to be a waste of time, so always set goals that are challenging. Considering the example above, you would need to consider if this role fits in with the current professional climate?

Timely goals

Goal setting can be unsystematic, sporadic and disorganised and because of these goals will be forgotten, achievement of goals will not be measured and feedback will not occur into new goals. The major benefits of goal setting have therefore been lost. Be organised and regular in the way that you use goal planning simply by setting a timeframe for the goal, for example, by December 2013, 6 months, 12 months etc. Establishing a timeframe gives you an end point and clear targets. By not identifying a timeframe the commitment to the goal becomes too vague. It tends not to happen because there is no urgency to start. In addition, too many un-prioritised goals may be set, leading to a feeling of overload. Remember that you deserve time to relax and enjoy being human.

Once you have identified your goals and objectives, you would need to look at how you will set out to achieve them. Action planning is a logical sequence with a central focus to specific areas of development/change. This will identify what you are going to do, how you are going to do it, by when and in what order. This will involve identifying explicitly all components.

Often, action plans can be limited and lack the specific detail that is needed to produce a realistic, feasible plan that will enable success. It is therefore important to set individual actions that are specific to each objective. This has two purposes:

1.   It ensures that all areas of required action have been taken into account
2.   It breaks the achievement process down into manageable chunks

When setting your actions it is important to use verbs to describe what you intend to do, such as 'read', 'practice', 'implement' etc. It is also important to identify a range of ways to achieve your objectives and cross reference to the factors identified in your SWOT analysis. This will help to maximise those factors (strengths and opportunities) and will help you progress and minimise or neutralise factors (weaknesses and threats) that will hinder your progress (Nicklin and Kenworthy, 2000) as these will certainly influence your action plan.

Regardless of how good an action plan is, there are many potential reasons that prevent actions from happening. Such barriers include tasks that can be too difficult, have too many objectives or the lack of mechanisms for on-going monitoring of action plan outcomes. Breaking down the tasks, identifying actions, identifying resources and identifying adequate time to complete can help you to succeed. Effective action planning can influence your personal and professional development and as a cyclical process it will enable further developments.

When recognizing resources to support your actions you will need to consider people, time, space and equipment. For example, if you are undertaking a course the resources you could access would be lecturers, library staff, books, journals, computer, and internet and cost, of course, if you are self-funding etc. These are opportunities that you could use identified in your SWOT analysis.

Table 9.2 illustrates an action plan that is directly linked to the SWOT analysis in Box 9.1. As you will see, the goal and action plan directly relate to the areas identified in each section of the SWOT analysis that will make the goals and action plan successfully achieved.

Discussion point

Consider your personal and professional development. If you are a newly qualified paramedic or nurse, reflect on your pre-registration training and identify your development for the next 12 months. What skills are you good at? What gaps in your knowledge and skills do you need to address? How you will set about reducing those gaps? How long will this take? Think through your career and where you would like to be in 3 years' time, how will you achieve your ambitions? Now think how you are going to record that to start your professional journey.

Organising your portfolio

Portfolios whether it is personal, educational or professional can take many forms. Compilations of hard-copy documents are probably the most familiar portfolio format; however, developments in knowledge, information and learning technologies have prompted the emergence of digital or electronic portfolios, referred to as 'e Portfolios' or 'webfolios'. Employers and/or professional organisations may provide you with a portfolio that will be divided into required sections and may include a range of templates for self-assessments, curriculum vitae, reflections etc. This will provide you with some direction and guidance; however, you may choose to develop your own portfolio. This will enable you to diversify and be creative to allow you to personalise your portfolio giving you greater autonomy and ownership of your development and how this is demonstrated. Whether you compile your information electronically or in a binder folder, a neat professional product is the objective. This means that materials should be typed, sections should be labelled and a table of contents should be prepared and your name and contact information should be easy to find. It is important to include your CV in a portfolio, which can be placed in the beginning.

When starting your portfolio, it may seem a daunting task at first as it can be difficult to know where to start and what evidence to use. It would seem common sense to start putting in your CV, certificates of courses, workshops, testimonials, reflections and whatever other pieces of paper you can

Table 9.2 Example of action plan with cross referencing (Evidence No. 4.2)

	Goal: To become an effective mentor by April 2013				
Specific goals/objectives	**Actions**	**Resources**	**Evidence used**	**Achieved by**	**X-ref**
1. To complete a university mentorship course	To find locally available courses To attend sessions on module To complete all formative assessments To complete all summative assessments To secure funding for course	University prospectus Internet Module tutors Funding from employer Library Study skills sessions Paramedic students Clinical practice	Certificate of completion	April 2012	5a, 6a, 7b, 9c, 10a
2. To gain experience of mentor role	To shadow mentors in practice To mentor students in practice To read theory of mentor role and responsibilities To be supervised by experienced mentors to ensure reliability of assessing students	Mentor Clinical practice Paramedic student(s) Books, journals	Feedback from students Feedback from mentors Reflective writing	30.07.12 30.07.12 30.08.12	5a, 7c, 9c 5a, 7c, 9c 5a, 7c, 9c
3. To successfully mentor three students	To review the students competency documents To work and supervise student(s) for the duration of the practice placement To prepare and deliver structured teaching sessions for specific skills To liaise with paramedic course lecturers To liaise with mentors for advise To obtain feedback from students To arrange annual appraisal	Course competency documents Lecturers Mentors Paramedic students Evaluation forms Facilities for teaching (training school)	Written evaluation from students Peer review from mentor(s) Reflective writing Annual appraisal documentation	30.01.13 11a 30.01.13 30.02.13 25.02.13	5a, 7c, 9c 5a, 7c, 11a 5a, 7c, 9c 7c, 9c, 11a

use to fill out your portfolio and add other documents when completed. When compiling your portfolio you need to consider the following:

- Conceptualise how you will use your portfolio
- How you will make reference to your portfolio
- Your regulatory body standards for re-registration
- Types of evidence required

Table 9.3 provides an example of three types of categories and evidence for each category. This list is not exhaustive and you will need to filter your evidence to ensure it meets the aims and objectives of your personal and professional development and shows learning and progression. It is important to note that portfolios should not be cluttered with copies of articles, leaflets, policies or procedures without some reason or annotation on them to explain their relevance to practice.

Options are to put your portfolio in chronological order or in sections using section dividers. This will make it easy to insert and locate the evidence you have included. Within your sections of your portfolio, you would need to label your evidence individually so that it can easily be located. Tables 9.2 and 9.3 have been individually labelled to illustrate this or you

Table 9.3   Categories and types of evidence

Categories of evidence	Types of evidence
Self-assessment	SWOT analysis Goal setting, action plans
Feedback from others	Testimonials, clinical supervision records Letters from patients, commendations Feedback from tutors Appraisal documentation Peer reviews Witness statements
Evidence of achievement	Certificates of attendance to workshops, study events, conferences etc. Certificates of achievement Reflective writings Written case studies Competency documents Critical case analysis Job description Annotated bibliographies Teaching sessions undertaken List of committees and documentation of participation in meetings (e.g. minutes from those meetings) Publications Conference presentations

could simply use handwritten labelled stickers. It might also be necessary to cross reference your evidence to other sections of your portfolio to verify claims and link a piece of work to another piece of work with related interests.

Cross referencing which is abbreviated as x-ref or xref is simply relating information from one source to another to make connections. For instance, index pages in books are cross referencing as this tells you the page number(s) of the specific subject. There are several ways to use cross referencing and if you review the action plan in Table 9.2 which illustrates one method of cross referencing the evidence within a portfolio. Related pieces of work can be in more than one section (as illustrated in Table 9.3).

It is likely that you will achieve other skills and/or competences in your work as illustrated in Box 9.2. As you will see from this illustration, all the skills have a different symbol and to cross reference these skills you just simply add the symbol to the evidence you have used (Box 9.3). For example, if you reflect on an incident in practice that demonstrates how you used effective communication skills to obtain a history from a patient whose first language is German, then you would insert the appropriate symbol on your evidence. Other commonly used methods are to:

- include on the contents page
- add a separate page or table to show how cross referencing has been applied
- use of headers or footnotes at the end of your evidence, for example:
  Further evidence to demonstrate achievement of this skill is found in
  Section 5: Evidence No. 5.1, 5.2 and 5.3
  Section 10: Evidence No. 4.2, 5.3, 6.2 and 10b

Whichever method of organisational systems to structure and cross reference your portfolio contents you would need to make this clear and state this as part of your introduction. Just remember that as the owner of your

---

Box 9.2   Example of portfolio structure

Section 1	Portfolio explanation – details and purpose of portfolio
Section 2	Personal details – curriculum vitae and/or personal statement
Section 3	Job descriptions
Section 4	Self-assessments
Section 5	Continuing professional development
Section 6	Continuing professional education
Section 7	Reflective practice
Section 8	Evidence based practice
Section 9	Teaching experience
Section 10	Certificates of attendance and/or achievement
Section 11	Testimonials

Box 9.3   Symbol coding of skills to cross reference with evidence

Core Skills

Basic airway skills

Advanced airway skills

Patient assessment skills

Drug administration

Professional accountability

Transferable Skills

Communication skills

Leadership skills

Management skills

Evidence based practice

Reflective practice

Problem solving

portfolio, you will develop your own structure and feel comfortable and confident with the knowledge that you can locate the evidence; yet, this may not be the case to another reader. Your portfolio must make sense to the viewer with minimal guidance. To ensure that your portfolio is easy to navigate, ask a colleague to review this.

Summary

This chapter has provided a brief overview of the political agenda that has had a major influence to support and drive forward the concept of life-long learning and CPD which is now an integral part of everyday professional practice for all individuals working in healthcare. Service users can expect to receive a high quality standard of care delivered by competent and knowledgeable healthcare practitioners. The regulatory body have defined standards to ensure that registrants practice safely, legally and competently (NMC, 2008; HCPC, 2012a, c) and all registrants have to formally declare they are fit to practice and have met the standards for CPD (NMC, 2011; HCPC, 2012a) when renewing their registration. Qualified professionals need to understand that CPD is not about obtaining certificates of attendance to courses as this may only prove you attended the training event. It is important to think of CPD a daily part of professional practice as there are a range of opportunities available in a day to day practice as well as planned formal events. A good starting point when planning your CPD is to identify areas for development and the importance of self-assessment cannot be over emphasised. This will help you to build the foundations for your development and progression. There is a plethora of self-assessment tools available to use and this chapter has included the use of a SWOT analysis and goal setting as a starting point. These are very simple and easy to use tools, but as you progress and become familiar with self-assessment you may want to broaden your horizons and experiment others that are most suitable for you.

The HCPC (2012c) and NMC (2008) standards place the responsibility of individuals to demonstrate they undertake CPD by maintaining a written record through the use of portfolios. A professional portfolio will demonstrate progression and development of learning from a cross section of opportunities; however, they are not easy to construct initially as it is difficult to know what evidence is required, what is relevant and/or irrelevant and what is essential to potential reviewers. Following the practical guidance given, this will enable you to effectively self-evaluate and plan your learning and developmental activities, identify CPD opportunities, choose the appropriate evidence, and to structure your portfolio in a logical format. The benefits of a well-structured and organised portfolio is that it will demonstrate your ability to plan, organise and record your development; career progression; support claims for accreditation of prior learning; applying for new posts and renewal of registration.

References

Bandura, A. (1997) *Self-efficacy: The Exercise of Control*. Freeman, New York.

Baume, D. (2001) *A Briefing on Assessment and Portfolios Assessment Series No 6*. Learning and Teaching Support Network, York.

Benner, P. (1984) *From Novice to Expert. Excellence and Power in Clinical Nursing Practice*, Addison-Wesley Publishing, Menlo Park, California.

Boud, D. (1992) The use of self-assessment schedule in negotiated learning. *Studies in Higher Education*, **17**(2), 85–200.

Boud, D. (1995) *Enhancing Learning through Self-Assessment*. Routledge, New York.

Brown, R.A. (1992) *Portfolio Development and Profiling for Nurses*. Quay Publishing Ltd., Lancaster.

Cangelosi, P.R. (2008) Learning portfolios: Giving meaning to practice. *Nurse Educator*, **33**(3), 125–127.

Coffey, A. (2005) The clinical learning portfolio: A practice development experience in gerontological nursing. *International Journal of Older People Nursing in association with Journal of Clinical Nursing*, **14**(8b), 75–83.

Department of Health (1997) *The New NHS: Modern Dependable*. DH, London.

Department of Health (1999) *A First Class Service: quality in the new NHS*. DH, London.

Department of Health (2000) *The NHS Plan: a Plan for Investment. a Plan for Reform*. DH, London.

Department of Health (2004) *NHS Knowledge and Skills Framework (NHS KSF) and the development review process (October 2004)*. DH, London.

Draper, J. & Clark, L. (2007) Impact of continuing professional education on practice: The rhetoric and the reality. *Nurse Education Today*, **27**(6), 515–517.

Driessen, E., van de Vleuten, C., Scuwirth, L., van Tartwick, J. & Vermont, J. (2005) The use of qualitative criteria for portfolio assessment as an alternative to reliability evaluation: a case study. *Medical Education*, **39**(2), 214–220.

Falchikov, N. & Boud, D. (1989) Student self-assessment in higher education: a meta-analysis. *Review of Educational Research*, **59**(4), 395–430.

General Medical Council (2007) *The New Doctor*. General Medical Council, London.

Gopee, N. (2008) *Mentoring and Supervision in Healthcare*. Sage Publications, London.

Harris, S., Dolan, G. & Fairbairn, G. (2001) Reflecting on the use of student portfolios. *Nurse Education Today*, **21**(4), 278–286.

Health & Care Professions Council (2012a) *Continuing Professional Development and Your Registration*. HCPC, London.

Health & Care Professions Council (2012b) *Standards of Proficiency. Parmedics*. HCPC, London.

Health & Care Professions Council (2012c) *Standards of Conduct, Performance and Ethics*. HCPC, London.

Jasper, M.A. (1995). The potential of the professional portfolio for nursing. *Journal of Clinical Nursing*, 4(4), 249–255.

Knowles, M.S., Holton, Elwood F., III. & Swanson, R.A. (2005). *The Adult Learner*. Elsevier, London.

Locke, E.A., & Latham, G.P. (1990) *A Theory of Goal Setting and Task Performance*, Prentice Hall, Englewood Cliffs.

Mattheos, N.M.C., Nattestad, A., Falk-Nilsson, E. & Attström, R. (2004) The interactive examination: assessing students' self-assessment ability. *Medical Education*, 38(4), 378–389.

Nicklin, P. & Kenworthy, N. (2000) *Teaching and Assessing in Nursing Practice. An Experiential Approach*, 3rd edn Baillière Tindall, London.

Nixon, V. (2008) Assessment. In: *Portfolios in the Nursing Profession. Use in Assessment Professional Development* (ed. K. Norman), p. 23. Quay Books, London.

Nursing and Midwifery Council (2008) The Code. *Standards of Conduct, Performance and Ethics for Nurses and Midwives*. NMC, London.

Nursing and Midwifery Council (2011) *The Prep Handbook*. NMC, London

Rees, C., Shepherd, M. & Chamberlain, S. (2005) The utility of reflective portfolios as a method of assessing first year medical students' personal and professional development. *Reflective Practice*, 6(1), 3–14.

Royal College of Nursing (2007) *A Joint Statement on Continuing Professional Development for Health and Social Care Practitioners*. RCN, London.

Stoker, D. (1998) Assessment in Learning (in) Understanding assessment issues. *Nursing Times*, 90(11), Section 7 i–vii.

Zimmerman, B.J. (1998) Developing self-fulfilling cycles of academic regulation: An analysis of exemplary instructional models. In: *Self-regulated Learning: From Teaching to Self-reflective Practice* (eds D.H. Schunk & B.J. Zimmerman). Guilford Press, New York.

Index

Note: Page numbers followed by b, f, and t indicate text in box, figure and table respectively.

Professional Practice in Paramedic, Emergency and Urgent Care, First Edition. Edited by Val Nixon.
© 2013 John Wiley & Sons, Ltd. Published 2013 by John Wiley & Sons, Ltd.